ALWAYS L(
NUMBE

ALWAYS LOOK AFTER NUMBER TWO!

A GUIDE TO BETTER HEALTH THROUGH COLONIC IRRIGATION AND BOWEL CARE

GALINA IMRIE

Cartoon illustrations: Roy Nixon
Frezia Zarrat

Anatomical drawings: Maurice Imrie
Frezia Zarrat

Editing: Jane Smith
Jackie Harding

DTP: Cobalt Graphic Design

FOTHERBY PRESS 2006

Published by Fotherby Press in 2006
First printing: March 2006

The information contained in this book is for educational and health promotion purposes only. The principles described in this book are intended to enhance health rather than to diagnose or treat any disease or medical condition.

The content of this book is based upon sources that the author believes to be reliable. It is current as of January 2006.

Imrie, Galina

Always look after number two! A guide to better health through colonic irrigation and bowel care.

1. Self-help 2. Health and Beauty 3. Personal development

ISBN 10: 0-9552462-0-2
ISBN 13: 978-0-9552462-0-3

Printed and bound in England by
Antony Rowe Ltd, Chippenham, Wiltshire

To curious kids of all ages, who have never stopped asking questions about their bodies, and searching for answers.

Foreword

This is a book that was shouting out to be written.

It found Galina's ear; this happening, coupled with her energy and passion for the subject has produced her first book.

It is highly readable, and, no doubt, will stimulate the reader to think more of their own health in relation to their bowel habits.

There are few good books on the gastro-intestinal tract and its functions. The best, in my opinion, so far have been written by authors in the USA. This book has the makings of being a well thumbed piece of work, of interest to lay and professional readers alike.

Colon hydrotherapy is an ancient modality (colon lavage was first recorded 3,500 years ago). Now with modern, hygienic devices and fully disposable colonic treatment kits, as well as competent, professional consultants and therapists, colon hydrotherapy is an exciting modality.

In the UK it is within the field of Complimentary and Alternative Medicine (CAM). In China and Russia it is part of Integrative Medicine, as it should be in the West.

Several CAM modalities that were ridiculed by the conventional western medical fraternity not so long ago are now not only accepted, but adopted by allopathic medicine. The same will happen with colon hydrotherapy once it can produce medical evidence of its efficacy & worth by research. It badly needs benefactors to fund that research.

Dr James A Wiltsie MD, a medical doctor and an ardent

advocate of colon hydrotherapy, forewarned that: "Our knowledge of the normal and abnormal physiology of the colon and its pathology and management has not kept pace with that of many organs and systems of the body. As long as we continue to assume that the colon will take care of itself, just that long will we remain in complete ignorance of perhaps the most important source of ill health in the whole body."

Many individual colon hydrotherapists worldwide have, collectively, a huge resource of knowledge and experience.

We all need to share that resource openly, like Galina, for the good of the profession and for the benefit of our clients.

So, let us keep our minds open as well as our bowels and our clients' bowels.

Well done Galina. I look forward to your future work.

Allan Gray,

Colon Hydrotherapy Instructor,
Principal of the European College of Naturopathic Medicine (ECNM)

www.ecnm.org

The Health Benefits Of Colonics Are Just Too Good To Keep Quiet About

I sat down to read Number Two and realised that this is probably the most complete book on colonic irrigation and bowel health ever to be published. This book speaks to the health conscious and the curious, to the practitioner, the health professional and the patient. Within these pages, there is something to inspire anyone who has ever contemplated feeling healthier, happier and living a more energetic life.

As a naturopathic therapist I have dealt with the health of digestive systems and bowels for over ten years now. However, reading this book has reminded me yet again of the infinite wisdom of the human body. Galina has an easy, humorous and entertaining way of explaining human digestion and elimination, what can and does go wrong with it, and what can be done to make it all right again.

Naturopathic philosophy sees a healthy, functioning digestive system as the foundation of good health. This has always been the focal point of any treatment a naturopath will provide. In the modern world, where many of us are taking copious amounts of supplements and tonics, buying organic food and avoiding chemicals wherever we can, this book reminds us that it is the simple things, such as the body being able to eliminate daily wastes, that contribute hugely to our health and wellness.

In Sydney, Australia, I work with many practitioners and medical doctors that have found detoxification programs to be incredibly effective for their patients. When the gut and liver are working well and in harmony to eliminate wastes from the body, many otherwise 'untreatable' health conditions will disappear or be alleviated.

In the traditional naturopathic treatment this detoxification process has always been achieved through the use of dietary changes, herbal medicines and nutritional supplementation. In my experience, colonic irrigation treatments at certain stages of the detoxification process produce phenomenal results: programmes that may have taken two to six months can be achieved in as little as six weeks with the addition of colonics.

Patients report immediate results that keep them motivated and have them feeling fantastic and energised throughout the process. This supports Galina's observations that, in her experience, most people can achieve a higher level of health very quickly.

In her book Galina also provides sound and sensible advice on how to keep your body at its optimum level of health. She discusses the main elements of healthy living in everybody's life, including her own. Galina is living proof of the benefits of her knowledge and experience.

The astounding success of her treatment centre and day spa is testament to the number of people she has helped, and to the number of people whose health has improved so dramatically that they are not too embarrassed to tell their friends, families and colleagues to "go for a colonic": the health benefits are just too good to keep quiet about!

This book also speaks of the interesting and intimate connection between the bowel and human emotions - a well-known phenomenon in any science that works with people.

Naturopathically, we have always tried to clear the emotions to free the bowel. Galina's approach of clearing the bowels to free the emotions shows her sensitive insight into what she refers to as 'the language of the bowel'.

I thank Galina for her extensive research on this subject and for sharing her wisdom and experience with patients, sceptics and fellow practitioners. She should be commended for bringing 'the poo', that has been a 'taboo' subject in many healing circles, both medical and natural, into the mainstream. Now everybody can have a thorough understanding of the positive benefits colonic irrigation can bring to their health.

Reading this book has given me renewed passion for the healing arts and has confirmed my faith in the human body, reminding me that, no matter what the 21st century throws at us, there is always a path back to abundant health.

More often than not it is as simple as 'looking after number two'.

Yours in health,

Lara Coleman, ND, BSc
lcoleman@healthworld.com.au

CONTENTS

Working with the bowel is a privilege - it tells the stories of health and disease, body management and abuse, balanced nutrition and addictions. It does this all without using words, gestures or excuses about cruel parents, inner-city schools and uncaring peers.

Bowel eliminations reflect how we, here and now, take responsibility for our health, both physical and emotional. The bowel story is a great story, and there are many ways of telling it.

I thought a simple guide to colonic irrigation would be a good start. There are lots of myths and misconceptions surrounding this treatment, and virtually no information in print, especially in comparison to the vast literature covering massages, reflexology, homeopathy, herbal cleansing and other holistic disciplines.

This is probably one of the first modern books about colonics. I hope it will open the floodgate (no pun intended!). I am sure there will be more books, and that there will be others who will help the public to warm to the bowel and see the beauty and poetry in Quasimodo.

Disclaimer

The purpose of this book is to provide information and advice to those wondering how colon hydrotherapy could enhance their health and add life to their years.

It is based on my knowledge and experience as a detoxification practitioner, holistic colon hydrotherapist, massage therapist, thinker and teacher. My recommendations are not specific to you, they are general and they are designed to help you understand the connection between the different signs and symptoms that you can observe in your body. They are not a substitute for medical advice.

Acknowledgements

I am immensely grateful to my colleagues in Wellbeing Now, for sharing my convictions, for believing in bowel management through whole-person management and for integrating colonics into their holistic practices. Shoela Detsios, thank you for your amazing naturopathic knowledge, a great quest for health promotion and dry wit. Kim Verhoeven, thank you for being a daring, vulnerable and passionate practitioner. Thank you both for building, together with me and others, an amazing practice that has helped so many people.

Writing 'Number Two' would have been a lot more solitary, had it not been for Frezia Zaraat, my personal assistant, audio-typist, sounding board, person Friday and talented art student, who has helped illustrate this book.

The dry humour of Roy Nixon's cartoons has given the bowel story a new visual dimension that, I hope, will bring a smile or two to your face.

I am very grateful to Jane Smith for her extremely tactful editing and to Jackie Harding for the complete opposite.

I am also indebted to my mentors. There are many people I have learned from, but few stand out. I am especially grateful to the great personal development coach, Tony Robbins, for helping me to bring passion to every breath I take; Dr. Sanjay Chaudhuri, a visionary who has taught me to catch my thoughts, put them on paper and share them with others; and finally, Ernest Coates, a great Yogi and modern guru, who has shown me the way to grow my spiritual being by stretching me well past my physical boundaries. You taught me how not to break. I have learned to stand tall from all of you.

And finally, I am always, unreservedly, grateful to my husband Steve, who builds my dreams.

COLONICS IN A NUTSHELL

In a nutshell, colonics is about letting go.

COLONICS IN A NUTSHELL.....

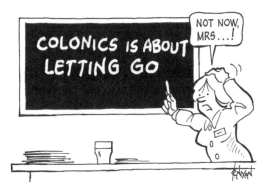

Few other treatments enable you to let go to such a great extent. Here you are, lying on the couch, water going in and out of your body, as you are watching your eliminations float past in the view tube, carried away by water, like a river after a flood.

Getting rid of the waste is a cathartic, purifying feeling; a kind of a cleansing ritual, which helps bring together the body and the spirit in a desire for better health.

Sometimes you may feel mild discomfort or a cramp, as the bowel struggles to get vintage wastes out. Often you feel a great, overpowering urge to evacuate, and it is during these evacuations that you resolve to make positive changes in the way you treat yourself.

Sometimes you come to the colonics feeling numb and tired. As the process starts, you are suddenly overwhelmed by emotions, as your feelings, composted between layers of wastes, come out and demand acknowledgement. At times a good cry helps. It is a shame to let these emotions out through the back door - they need to be recognized for what they are and felt in every cell of the awakened body.

Going for a colonic involves a certain degree of honesty and recognition that you need to change: at the end of the day, colonics is not a facial. It is a great first step on the road of self-improvement through action and knowledge, of self-discovery through purification, and of physical cleansing through waste management.

Thank you for reading this book. Whether you are driven by curiosity or you want an action plan, I hope I will be able to help you along the way. Your journey is about to begin - have a good one!

INTRODUCTION

Is this book for me?

You are probably wondering if this book is for you. The broad answer is 'yes' - if you have ever had an unsatisfactory bowel movement, and you wondered why, this book may help you find the clues. If you have ever wanted to understand how a slice of pizza turns into 40 grams of brown matter, then read on.

If you have considered colonic irrigation, but were disappointed by the scarcity of published materials, I hope this book will go some way towards satisfying your curiosity and desire to understand how the treatment works and how you can benefit from it.

If you have never considered colonics, and this book has attracted your attention by its unconventional title or subject matter, read it as you would read any other story - for pleasure, for fun or to pass the time.

There is a chance that the underlying idea of this book - health improvements through bowel movements - may grow on you and help you gain a better quality of life. And if it does not, I hope you will have a good time just immersing yourself in the bizarre workings of someone else's mind.

If you are a medical professional who is puzzled by the fact that colonic treatments are becoming more and more popular, the stories of real people in this book may help you understand why. Even if you feel strongly that these people are duped, misguided and fooled, you will see that they feel better, have a better connection with the workings of their bodies and a better understanding of the causal links between ingestion, digestion, absorption, assimilation and elimination than they otherwise would have. If nothing else, their success stories deserve some attention from a medical practitioner.

If you feel bloated, constipated, sluggish, tired and worn out, and your complaints are being routinely dismissed by your doctor, who does not understand why you won't just take a laxative or two and get on with it, then this book is definitely for you. It will open another door that you did not know existed.

You just might decide to take the first step towards your health management through bowel cleansing and colonics. This is up to you and I will be really happy if you do. I hope the information contained in this book will help you find a good holistic practitioner of colonics who will guide you towards better health.

If you are student of colonics, then read this book as a shortcut to understanding why people will come to you, what they want, and how they expect you to help them - and rise to the challenge.

If you are a colon hydrotherapist, I hope this book will give you some new ideas and will inspire you to carry on. I hope it will show you the great value of the work you already do, and other ways of helping large numbers of people and enhancing your business.

If you are a sceptic who has decided to read this book to prove me wrong, I hope that I won't make it easy for you. This book is not about who is right and who is wrong, it is about helping ordinary people to achieve extraordinary health without drugs. Please bear this in mind and be fair.

Let me take you on a journey

I would like to take you on an interesting journey.

In Part One of this book I explain the basics of the digestive system, how it works and how you can start reading the signs and signals that the body sends to you when it needs to let you know how it feels. Not everyone can be a mind reader, but all of us can develop some very simple 'body-reading' techniques and use them on a daily basis.

From then on, we'll move round in circles.

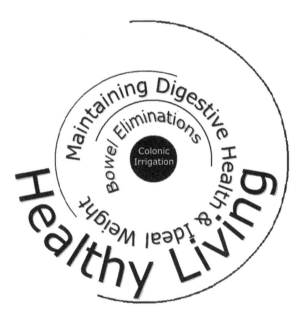

Part Two is the main reason why you decided to read this book. It is a guide to colonic irrigation. In this part you will, I hope, learn everything you need to know to make an informed decision about colonics: history of the colonic tradition; the colonic process and the results that you can achieve by having colonic irrigation treatments. You will also find out how to choose colonic irrigation equipment and the right colon hydrotherapist, what you need to know about the procedure and what are the related treatments that can enhance the effect of your colonic.

After reading this part, you should also be able to assess the standards of the practice you have chosen and to ask informed questions about the equipment and the materials used for your treatments.

It will then be time to have a glimpse of the bigger picture, which is considered in Part Three.

Part Three is all about the poo - how our eliminations are formed, how much is good enough, how to improve your eliminations, how to check if your bowel is working properly and what your 'poo' should ideally look like. I will also give you some guidelines on paying attention to certain signs in your eliminations that might tell you what is going on in your body, and what challenges your digestive system encounters on a daily basis.

We will then move on to Part Four which I have dedicated to healthy eating. I will map out some simple steps you can take to enhance your health and digestion and improve your weight management. These steps are easy and logical. They reflect common sense. But when you put them together you will be able to create a system of your daily nutrition that will help you choose the right foods, eat them properly and ensure you maximize your absorption of the nutrients contained within them.

From healthy eating we will progress to healthy living in Part Five. We will talk about healthy breathing, hydration, nourishing emotion, maintaining a higher energy level by cleansing the lymphatic system, exercise, eating living foods, and cleansing the body. These are the main elements of healthy living that I believe would be of benefit to every single one of us.

The Epilogue is about me. Every time I read a self-help book, I wonder how the author uses the advice and knowledge contained within it. I think I walk my talk: that is why I have included a short section on how I have arrived at, in short, 'being me'.

The client quotations used in this book are genuine. I have removed or changed clients' names, for obvious reasons of confidentiality. Otherwise, the thoughts that they put on paper are presented virtually verbatim.

There are a few short appendices at the end of the book: a short list of some very good books, that I have read at different stages of my learning, and that have helped me shape my idea of health; the colon hydrotherapy questionnaire that we use in Wellbeing Now (www.wellbeingnow.co.uk), and useful web addresses, including those of colon hydrotherapy practitioners' associations, schools, nutritionists and educators.

I have also included a description of an exercise routine that can help you relax, get rid of toxins, reduce bloatedness and manage stress.

You can e-mail your comments through the website, www.colonicbook.com, or write to Wellbeing Now, 17 North Town Road, Maidenhead, Berkshire, SL6 7JQ.

PART ONE

THE BASICS OF THE DIGESTIVE SYSTEM

THE INS AND OUTS OF THE DIGESTIVE SYSTEM.....

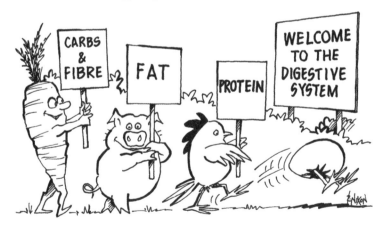

PART ONE: THE BASICS OF THE DIGESTIVE SYSTEM

Main terms explained

The ins and outs of the digestive system

The bowel is our second brain

The bowel is a creature of habit

Summary: your road map to the basics of the digestive system

Main terms explained

Absorption - *Absorption is the second stage of* **digestion,** *after* **ingestion.** *Absorption means that food, already broken down into nutrients, is able to cross the barrier between the sealed digestive system and the blood stream. In order to be absorbed properly, nutrients need to be in a form that is recognizable to human cells.*

Assimilation - *Occurs following* **absorption,** *when nutrients enter human cells and turn into components similar to those that human cells already possess.*

Autointoxication - *A term that is used to describe the re-absorption of gut toxins back into the blood stream. The term I prefer is* **leaky gut syndrome***.*

Bowel - *A term that may mean large or small intestine. In this book it is used to mean the large intestine. See also '***Colon'** *and '***Gut'***.*

Candida - *There are hundreds of forms of Candida, a yeast-like fungus that is naturally present everywhere on the planet. Candida albicans, the best-known version of Candida, is a form of* **gut dysbiosis** *(imbalance of gut bacteria), an excessive fermentation of sugars that can be caused by dietary imbalances and malnutrition, as well as by low emotional and immune states.*

Colon - *Another name for the* **large intestine** *or* **bowel***.*

Colon hydrotherapy - *Also called colonic irrigation or high colonic, this is a term used to describe the process of cleansing the* **large intestine, bowel** *or the* **gut** *with water, which is introduced into the bowel through the anal opening.*

Colonic irrigation - See Colon hydrotherapy.

Digestion - *The process by which food is dissolved and broken down so that it can be absorbed by the cells of an organism and used to maintain the vital bodily functions.*

Digestive system - *A system in humans and other animals that enables digestion to take place. In humans, **digestive tract** is a long tube, comprising the mouth, oesophagus, stomach, small intestine, large intestine, rectum and anus. **Digestive system** support network also includes the liver, pancreas, spleen, gall bladder and the glands of the oral cavity.*

Dysbiosis - *An imbalance of micro-organisms in the digestive tract. Virtually every digestive disease has dysbiosis as its underlying cause. Dysbiosis can cause intolerances, Candida infections, indigestion and bloating, discomfort, headaches and other digestive health complaints.*

Elimination - *The final stage of **digestion**. It is the clean-up and removal of wastes and non-nutrients that are incompatible with our living cells and therefore can't be assimilated and used by the body.*

Enema - *A device used to introduce water through the anal opening into the rectum and descending colon to clear out the waste from these areas. The difference between the enema and the colonic is that the enema clears only a small section of the large intestine, whereas the colon hydrotherapy treatment can clear most of it.*

Enteric nervous system - *Located in the intestines, is the 'brain' that our gut uses to run the whole digestive process.*

Fermentation - *Chemical conversion of carbohydrates and fibre into simpler compounds by the action of enzymes, which are produced by micro-organisms such as yeasts and bacteria residing in the large intestine (see also **Gut bacteria**). Traditionally the term 'fermentation' is used, in relation to stools formation, to denote a bowel-friendly process. See also **Putrefaction**.*

Gut - *A general term which is used to mean **large** and **small intestine**, or the **bowel**.*

Gut bacteria - *Organisms that live in the large intestine, and to a lesser extent in the small intestine. Their main functions are to process wastes and to help the elimination process. Gut bacteria can be divided into several groups.*

> **Commensals** - *Commensal (from the Latin for 'eating at the same table') bacteria live in our gut, use it as their home and help some aspects of the eliminative function of the general health maintenance.*

> **Pathogenic** - *Pathogenic bacteria inhibit eliminative function, and cause **dysbiosis**.*

> **Probiotic** - *Probiotic bacteria actively support the eliminative function.*

> **Symbiotic** - *Symbiotic bacteria help some aspects of the eliminative function. Also see **Commensals**.*

Some bacteria can be commensal, symbiotic or pathogenic depending on our lifestyle, nutritional choices and the condition of our immune system.

Ingestion - The first stage of taking the food into the body, which initiates **digestion**.

Intestinal flora - Another term for **gut bacteria**.

Large Intestine - The part of the intestine where elimination and some assimilation take place. Other names for the large intestine are the **colon**, the large bowel and the gut.

Leaky gut syndrome - A combination of symptoms that can include bloating, indigestion, abdominal pain, constipation, diarrhoea and other digestive complaints caused by increased gut permeability. This means that the seal between the bowel and the rest of the body is breached, which enables toxins to penetrate the gut wall and get reabsorbed into the blood stream. Leaky gut or gut permeability has a negative effect on all other organs and systems of the body.

Malabsorption - Occurs when the body is unable to break down food into nutrients that can be assimilated by cells. It can be caused, among other factors, by malnutrition, shortage of stomach acid, insufficient activity of digestive enzymes or the presence of toxins in the body.

Neurotransmitter - Neurotransmitters and receptors are main components of the enteric nervous system, the gut's 'think tank'. They have a similar function to the factors that ensure the process of thinking in our brain.

Parasite - Organisms that live inside the host, use the host and negatively affect the host's function. Humans suffer mostly from single-cell parasites (microparasites) and worms. Parasites mainly live in the digestive tract, but sometimes they can *also invade muscles or connective tissue.*

*> **Putrefaction** - Decomposition of proteins. In relation to bowel health, this term is commonly used to denote the decay of protein and fat matter in the gut, which has a negative impact on health, such as constipation, diarrhoea and bloatedness. See also* **Fermentation***.*

*> **Serotonin** - The neurotransmitter that determines, to a very large extent, our mood. It is sometimes described as the happiness factor. 95% of the serotonin that exists in our body is produced, stored and used in the* **large intestine***.*

*> **Small Intestine** - A section of the intestines where absorption and assimilation take place. Small intestine consists of the duodenum, the jejunum, and the ileum.*

The ins and outs of the digestive system

Human digestion is an enormous subject, and many great books have been written about it.

I will focus only on the most basic points that everyone should be aware of. Here they are, in a nutshell.

Food groups

The food we eat and the liquids we drink contain starches or carbohydrates, proteins and fats, fibre, enzymes, vitamins and minerals.

Starches or carbohydrates are the main components of grains, fruit and vegetables. Proteins are contained in animal food (anything that had parents is, broadly speaking, a protein),

THE HUMAN DIGESTIVE SYSTEM

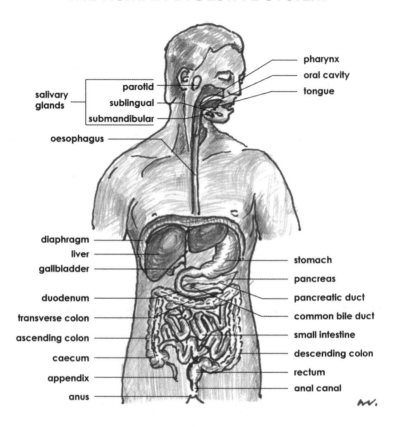

as well as in beans, pulses and sea vegetables. Fats are contained in protein-rich foods as well as in oils, grains, seeds and nuts.

Alcohol is a product of fermentation of carbohydrates. It is contained in fermented products - wines and spirits - as well as (in very small quantities) yoghurts, tofu and sauerkraut (yes, you can drive if you have had natural yoghurt - it is only 0.8% alcohol or less).

Carbohydrates, alcohols, proteins and fats are the food groups that have calories (Kcal). Carbohydrates have 4 Kcal per gram, proteins have 4, alcohol has 7 and fats have 9. Calories in food are the units of energy required by the body. This is the energy that enables all body processes to take place.

Fruit, vegetables and grains also contain insoluble fibre, which the body does not break down but which it uses to mop up wastes. Fats and proteins do not contain any fibre at all.

Fresh food contains enzymes - catalysts of the digestive processes. All food groups contain vitamins and minerals, which we need for the healthy functioning of all our organs.

Insoluble fibre has some calories (although they can't be used by the body), whereas enzymes, vitamins and minerals do not contain calories at all.

Processed foods have additives - chemical dyes, preservatives and other components that the food industry uses as taste enhancers or in order to extend the shelf life of the food and make it look pretty. Although the body absorbs some of them, it is unable to assimilate them or use them in any other meaningful way.

A complicated tube

The body requires carbohydrates to produce energy. Proteins are used by the body for rebuilding and maintaining healthy cells and bones as well as the blood and lymphatic systems. Fats are very important for the work of neurotransmitters: they help the assimilation of vitamins and other nutrients and are

THE INS AND OUTS OF THE DIGESTIVE SYSTEM.....

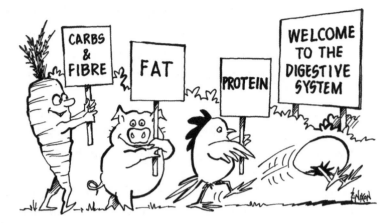

also used by the body as a long-term energy store, which it can call upon when it's running low on carbohydrates.

All these nutrients are being ingested, digested, absorbed, assimilated and eliminated in the digestive tract. The digestive tract is a long tube which starts in the mouth and ends in the anus. It is a sealed system, which basically means that the food we eat can communicate directly only with the mouth, the oesophagus, the stomach, the small intestine and the large intestine, but not with any other organs.

Communication between food and such organs as the liver, kidney, heart, brain etc is indirect. After the food is broken down into its constituent parts, blood delivers these constituents to the organs to enable them to function properly.

One exception to this rule is alcohol. Alcohol is the ultimate non-nutrient that contains calories but no vitamins or minerals. It goes straight into the blood, bypassing the whole digestive process, hitting the liver before you have finished the first glass, and the brain soon afterwards.

Generally, we can now see why some doctors believe that humans are nothing but a complicated tube. Everything we are able to do, our great thought processes, our great achievements, our great sporting conquests, are, in effect, the result of the body having enough carbon to do the job right, and the mind focusing on the achievement.

Stages of digestion

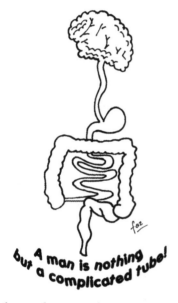

but a man is nothing a complicated tube!

Digestion begins in the mouth. When we chew, we start breaking up carbohydrates and warming up the chewed food, while also adding moisture to proteins and fats, preparing them for further processing. Saliva in the mouth also acts as a mild antiseptic agent, destroying some of the undesirable bacteria and parasites that we ingest with food.

Then the food passes down the oesophagus into the stomach. The stomach has two main functions: it acts as the chamber where proteins get broken down, and as a bacteria-zapping device, the stomach acid destroying undesirable organisms that have survived the saliva test in the mouth. It is a very acidic environment.

Then food goes into the small intestine, which is very long: about 3.5 times your height. It accounts for about 75 per cent of the whole length of the digestive tract. This is where food is broken down further, nutrients are absorbed so that they can be delivered to our internal organs and assimilated, and the wastes, insoluble fibre and other components that can't be assimilated are shunted into the large intestine by peristaltic movements of the intestinal wall.

The main functions of the large intestine are to absorb water and eliminate wastes. It also manufactures some vitamins and important neurotransmitters such as serotonin, and provides immune support for the rest of the body. You will learn more about the functions of the large intestine in Parts Two and Three of this book, when we look more closely at bowel eliminations.

Finally the wastes are eliminated through the rectum and anus.

.....OUR GREAT ACHIEVEMENTS, OUR GREAT SPORTING CONQUESTS ARE, IN EFFECT, THE RESULTS OF THE BODY HAVING ENOUGH CARBON TO DO THE JOB RIGHT......

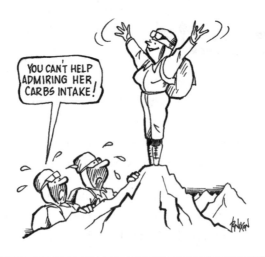

The bowel is our second brain

There are a few interesting things that we need to remember about the bowel. The whole of the digestive system works fairly independently from the central nervous system.

The main function of the central nervous system is to run all of the conscious processes in our body over which we have control, such as moving our muscles, walking, talking, blinking, yawning etc.

Of all digestive processes, the only ones over which we have voluntary control are the process of chewing and swallowing - the initial digestive events - and the opening of our external anal sphincter to allow the body to eliminate the wastes - the final digestive event.

After we have swallowed, we have virtually no control over the digestive and eliminative process until our brain is called upon to consciously open the anal sphincter. The whole process of digestion and elimination project is controlled routinely by our enteric nervous system, which is often described as the second brain.

On a daily basis, it communicates feelings of hunger and satiety to the head brain. In emergencies, when something goes seriously wrong, it also communicates negative feelings to the brain, such as the urge to vomit, abdominal pain, nausea and other SOS signals that the bowel needs to resort to when it requires team work to eliminate an offending substance from the body. When an emergency occurs, it asks the head brain to mobilize other internal organs to help it accomplish the process of cleaning-up.

Our head brain normally leaves the bowel alone, having a direct effect on the bowel only in times of stress. Stress requires

..... IN EMERGENCIES IT (THE ENTERIC NERVOUS SYSTEM) ALSO COMMUNICATES TO THE BRAIN NEGATIVE FEELINGS WHEN SOMETHING GOES SERIOUSLY WRONG : THESE ARE THE URGE TO VOMIT, ABDOMINAL PAIN, NAUSEA AND OTHER SOS SIGNALS .....

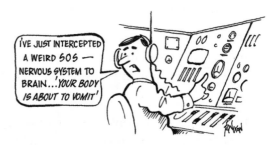

increased oxygen consumption by such important organs as the brain itself, the heart and the liver, so some of the blood will have to be diverted from the bowel to these organs, and the digestive processes will slow down.

The enteric nervous system also establishes communications between some 200 to 500 different organisms that inhabit the bowel and puts in place the system of checks and balances that, in a healthy body, ensure healthy co-existence amongst all the creatures in the gut zoo.

If you are still not convinced that the bowel has 'emotions', remember how you feel before an important event, such as an exam or a date: you have butterflies in your stomach, you have a 'gut feeling' about the outcome, and so on.

These simple things should help you understand that the bowel is not just a massive waste dump. In fact, it is anything but! 95% of the serotonin (the mood-regulating neurotransmitter) is manufactured in the bowel.

The bowel also contains a spread-out immune system that

helps the rest of the body to stay healthy.

There is a lot of research on the connection between the physiology and psychology of the bowel. 'The Second Brain' by Michael D. Gershon, M.D. (HarperCollins 2003) is the book that I have found invaluable and inspiring.

The bowel is a creature of habit

Our life has changed

Life in the twenty-first century is very different from life 150 years ago, when the main focus for most people was on staying close to the clan or tribe, mating with someone from the same peer group, or at the very least from the same culture and with the same conditioning, having a family, being faithful and having a rewarding career.

Basically, life was about being monogamous, both in relationships and in professions or careers. At least, that is what life had in store for most people.

Today, priorities have changed. The purposes of modern life are, broadly, to have multiple challenges, to experience different adventures, cultures and rituals, and only afterwards do all the 'boring adult things' such as like mating and procreating.

People want to have fun. They want to change careers; they want to change jobs, continents, places to live and relationships. Even as recently as 100 years ago people between the ages of 20 and 30 were already intending on finding a mate and settling down; now we engage in personal development, go scuba diving, climbing, trekking, working or travelling around the world instead.

As a result, the whole 'I'm here for a purpose' part of life is delayed until 35 and 45 years of age - when we eventually decide to settle down and have a family.

What we need to remember when jet-setting around the world on our different adventures, changing jobs, changing relationships, putting ourselves through the stresses of our daily lives, is that the brain enjoys all that, but the bowel doesn't.

The bowel needs time to adjust

Unlike the brain, which thrives on new challenges, the bowel is a creature of habit that has been dragged, kicking and shouting, into the twenty-first century.

BOWEL CHASING THE BRAIN AROUND THE WORLD.....

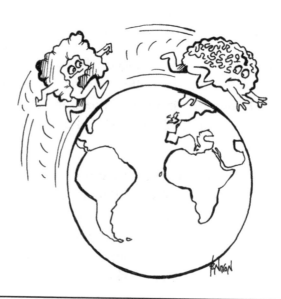

It takes a while for the bowel to establish a good working relationship with the ever-changing 200 to 500 colonies of different bacteria for which it serves as host. It also takes a while to adjust to the amount of fibre and protein or to make the best of the amount of water it is given. The gut does not change its habits overnight.

That is why when you go away on holiday sometimes the gut shuts down for a few days - it needs to re-adjust to the different food and water. Quite a few people find that their bowel movements change every time they change their water supply. To an extent, this is natural: it just means that the bowel has noticed.

So you shouldn't be too surprised that if one day you decided to give up your goo and glue diet and become a raw food vegan, your bowel movements would get worse and you would feel queasy, sluggish and disorientated for a while. After all, you have broken a habit of a lifetime.

If you wish to make substantial changes to your health, try to introduce these changes gradually.

You can start by eating more natural foods, less processed foods, replacing your pasta dishes with brown rice, barley or quinoa with roasted vegetables, replacing your sandwiches with a soup and salad, and increasing the amount of water that you drink. Slowly but surely, all these things will help you generate a happier bowel movement.

When you go away on holiday, make sure that whatever you eat looks freshly cooked, if you are used to cooked foods, or clean and freshly cut if you are used to salads. Make sure you drink bottled water and you don't have ice in your drinks, because in most places tap water is used to make ice.

Summary: your road map to the basics of the digestive system

- Carbohydrates or starches produce energy for the body.

- Proteins maintain and rebuild the cells of the body.

- Fats help the function of neurotransmitters and the assimilation of vitamins and are used as a long-term energy store.

- Chewing is an important part of the digestive process - the saliva begins to destroy harmful bacteria and chewing prepares the food for further processing.

- Once food has been swallowed we have no control over the digestive process until we need to eliminate the wastes. The gut communicates the feeling of hunger and the feeling of satiety to the brain; but in emergencies it communicates negative feelings, asking the brain to mobilize other organs in the body for help.

- The brain only has a direct effect on the bowel in times of stress - increased oxygen is needed for the brain and other important organs, and therefore the whole digestive process is slowed down.

- The bowel is not just a massive waste dump; it produces serotonin and also contains a spread-out immune system that supports the rest of the body.

- The brain thrives on new challenges, but the bowel is a creature of habit. The bowel needs to establish a good relationship amongst 200 to 500 different bacterial colonies, and takes a while to adjust to making the best out of the nutrients and water that it receives.

PART TWO

A GUIDE TO COLONIC IRRIGATION

DEHYDRATION . . . . .

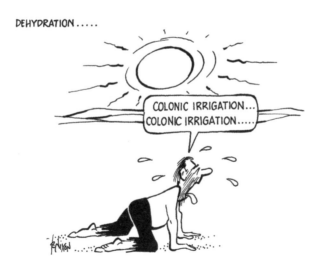

PART TWO: A GUIDE TO COLONIC IRRIGATION

Why colon cleansing is important in the modern world

A brief history of colon hydrotherapy

The seven Rs of colon hydrotherapy

Colon hydrotherapy and you

Main types of colonic equipment

Finding your colon hydrotherapist

Treatment procedure and commonly asked questions

Colonic irrigation and common digestive complaints

Colon hydrotherapy and related treatments

Summary: your road map to colonic irrigation

Why colon cleansing is important in the modern world

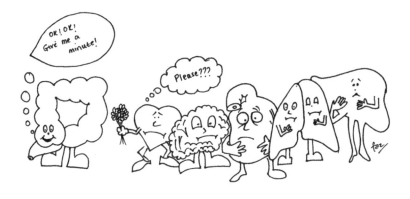

'One day the body's organs were having an argument as to which was the most important. The Brain was the first to gloat that without it the body couldn't think for itself and would do something really stupid and die.

The Heart disagreed, saying that without blood pumping around the body all the organs would suffocate from lack of oxygen. The Lungs said, 'Oh yeah and I provide the air for the rest of you guys so I'm the most important'. The Kidneys said that without them the body would poison itself and die. The Stomach said, 'Yeah but without me the body wouldn't be nourished'.

While the organs were arguing amongst themselves, the lowly Gut chimed in, 'Hey you guys what about me? Aren't I important?'

All the organs laughed and teased the poor little output device:' You're just a hole', they said, 'There is nothing to you...' and the poor little hole went into hiding saying: 'You're all mean, and to prove I'm the most important organ I'm going to hide and not do anything'.

They all continued laughing and eventually settled down for the night. The next morning, the Brain tried to wake up the body but didn't have enough energy to do so; the Heart felt a bit heavy and the Lungs were out of breath. The Stomach said he felt pretty congested and bloated, while the Kidneys complained that they couldn't keep up with the garbage the body was producing.

This went on for a few days until they remembered the lowly Gut.

'It was true', they all exclaimed. The poor little hole had clammed itself up in shame and affected the entire body!

'Okay...we give up! You are the most important organ in the body'.

And with that, the little hole gave out a huge sigh of relief, and the body was regular again.

We need to keep the colon clean

On a more serious note, we do need to make sure our colon is clean.

The human digestive system is a result of thousands of years of evolution. Digestive systems of people in most regions of world are designed to grind fresh hard foods, rich in fibre and nutrients, and low in calories, with an occasional feast on meat or fish.

The reality is that, with the exception of vegans and raw-food eaters, most of us consume our foods soft, cooked, or

Constipation is not really an issue in the animal kingdom

processed and chemically altered.

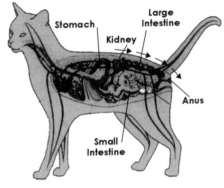

If you look at the design of the gut shown below, it is not hard to understand that it would work a lot more consistently if we were quadrupedal and the waste would not have to have the challenge of travelling up, across and then down. That's probably why constipation is not really an issue in the rest of the animal kingdom.

We do not have any reservations about brushing our teeth, washing our body, shampooing our hair, so grooming our second most intelligent organ should be just as, if not more, important!

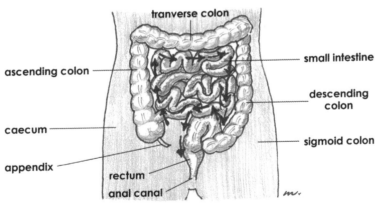

It's a long, long way from the caecum to the anus

Before we continue, there is one thing you need to be aware of: colon hydrotherapy is extremely effective, but it is not a silver bullet. Colonics is a great tool, and, as any tool, it needs to be used in accordance with its purpose.

The purpose of colon hydrotherapy is to improve and enhance your health and wellbeing primarily by improving the functioning of your digestive system. It needs to be used in combination with other tools, such as a healthy diet, exercise, bodywork, stress management, emotional growth, proper breathing, hydration and cleansing.

I've just finished my 2nd colonic but I think Galina suspects a different person came this time. Since my last visit two weeks ago I have completely changed my eating habits - low GI foods, no ready meals and lots more water.

This time the treatment was a breeze and I've managed to lose 6 lb in two weeks, without being hungry and not feeling like I'm on a diet. This was just the kick-start I need to begin a much healthier lifestyle. My diabetic consultant will be amazed when she sees my blood sugar results and that I have reduced my insulin by a third.

Now when I'm faced with something unhealthy, I ask myself whether I am prepared to suffer for it later. Nine times out of ten I'm not, but 1 out of 10, I'm human after all.

A brief history of colon hydrotherapy

Colon hydrotherapy is not a new procedure. Enemas and rituals involving the washing of the colon with water have been used since pagan times. The first record mentioning colon cleansing is an Egyptian medical papyrus dated as early as 1500 B.C. The Egyptians employed purgatives, enemas, diuretics, heat, steam and blood-letting to treat diverse diseases.

A BRIEF HISTORY OF COLON HYDROTHERAPY.....

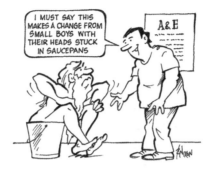

Ancient and modern tribes in the Amazon, Central Africa and remote parts of Asia have used river water for bowel cleansing, usually as part of magic-medical rites of passage performed by priests or shamans. Colon cleansing therapies were an important part of Taoist training regimens. These therapies still form one of the fundamental practices of the yoga teaching.

Hippocrates, Galen and Paracelsus, who are recognized as the founding fathers of Western medicine, described, practised and prescribed the use of enemas for colon cleansing.

An Enema

Both in Europe and in the USA, the popularity of colon cleansing treatments was remarkable in the early decades of the twentieth century, when colon irrigation equipment was commonly used by doctors practising in sanatoria (health spas) and hospitals. From the 1920s to the 1960s, the regular use of enemas was standard practice amongst most medical practitioners and they were implemented as common treatment in most hospitals.

With the rapid advancement of pharmaceutical approaches to treating various conditions, natural forms of healing, (including colon cleansing) had suffered a temporary setback. However, the pharmaceuticals have failed to deliver a neatly packaged 'pop and go' solution to annoying and tiring digestive complaints, such as malabsorption caused by underlying stress, constipation, bloating, recurrent yeast infections, dysbiosis, intestinal discomfort etc.

So, having travelled the full circle, we are back to natural healing. Now, having moved to the fringes of mainstream medical practice, colon hydrotherapy is fast becoming, yet again, one of the most popular holistic treatments.

By going for colon hydrotherapy you will find yourself in good company: Hollywood legend Mae West, Princess Diana and John Lennon were amongst the therapy's most famous adherents.

Anthony Robbins, one of the greatest personal development coaches of our time, uses colonics for himself, as a cleansing and health promotion therapy, and has become a great advocate of colonics as an important part of personal development and growth.

The seven Rs of colon hydrotherapy

Colon hydrotherapy is a great restorative treatment that gives a systemic boost to the body. The benefits of colon hydrotherapy all originate from removing stored wastes from the large intestine. Irrigating the gut with large amounts of water has many goals (see list below).

All these goals are interrelated, but it is only by looking at them more closely that we can get a truly three-dimensional picture of the physical, emotional and energetic changes that colonic irrigation achieves in the body.

> **THE SEVEN Rs OF COLON HYDROTHERAPY**
>
> 1. **Remove the wastes, irritants and allergy triggers.**
>
> 2. **Rehydrate the bowel.**
>
> 3. **Repair the gut wall.**
>
> 4. **Replace digestants and rebalance the bowel flora.**
>
> 5. **Rebuild the gut-brain connection**
>
> 6. **Restore the bowel function.**
>
> And finally....
>
> 7. **Re-educate the owner of the bowel.**

Remove the wastes, irritants and allergy triggers

In the process of colon hydrotherapy, wastes are removed from the bowel. The wastes are comprised of insoluble fibre, the red blood cells that have been used up by the body, cells of the stomach and the bowel lining, and indigestible materials including irritants and allergy triggers.

The pigment in red blood cells gives the stools its typical rusty-brown colour.

Everyone of us is aware, to a greater or lesser extent, that in the modern world we eat a lot of 'non-nutrients' that weren't designed to be eaten. These are pesticides that are used in the farming of grains and in the growing of fruit and vegetables, chemicals that are used to preserve our food and increase its shelf life, E-numbers, colorants and taste enhancers that are utilized in the manufacture of processed foods.

Food intolerances

Also, a significant number of people have poor tolerance of gluten, wheat, cows' milk and even of more innocent foods, such as tomatoes, onions and oranges for example. In addition to this, most people eat excessive amounts of animal protein, which the body can't break down and assimilate fully. In all honesty, a lot of people in the West eat far too much in general!

When we say that the body has poor tolerance of something, what does this actually mean? It means that it can't break that material down into useable components, absorb it, assimilate it and reuse it. So the body has no option but to try to eliminate the offending substances. Our most patient channel of elimination is the bowel, and sometimes it takes us a while to realize that something in our bowel isn't working properly.

When we try to eliminate excessive amounts of toxins through the skin, the skin breaks out and we develop skin eruptions. Elimination through our breath gives us bad breath, acid reflux and other symptoms that we notice immediately. The bowel, which is designed to store wastes for longer, is sometimes able to cope with irritants and allergy triggers for quite a while before reaching the critical point when we start suffering from bloatedness, constipation, diarrhoea, pain and discomfort.

One session of colon hydrotherapy probably won't eliminate everything that has been building up in the bowel over time. It can, nevertheless, start the process of further cleansing. With the appropriate diet and supplementation, you can continue having good quality elimination between treatments.

If you undertake colon hydrotherapy with a specific purpose of getting rid of certain allergic reactions or intolerances, it will probably make sense to have at least three treatments with short intervals between them, and monitor your body's reaction to them.

If you use colon hydrotherapy treatments to kick-start your knowledge of the body, and if you follow the proper nutritional advice and take your supplements, you will soon see that your periods of better health and wellbeing get longer between treatments. After three or four treatments, you will find the interval that is ideal for you and that enables you to maintain your health between the colonic treatments.

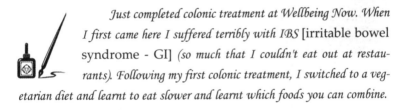

Just completed colonic treatment at Wellbeing Now. When I first came here I suffered terribly with IBS [irritable bowel syndrome - GI] *(so much that I couldn't eat out at restaurants). Following my first colonic treatment, I switched to a vegetarian diet and learnt to eat slower and learnt which foods you can combine.*

The 'Beauty breakfast' suggested was fantastic and I will continue to eat it even though I'm feeling much better. I changed my lifestyle slightly but the difference has been remarkable. I feel completely cured and will continue to keep an eye on what I eat. Thank you so much for sorting out an eight-year problem!

Rehydrate the bowel

A lot is written about people being chronically dehydrated in the modern world. Is it true? Or is it fiction? At the end of the day, we still function; we still survive. So how come we are chronically dehydrated?

There are three or four different reasons why people are a lot more dehydrated today than even one or two generations ago.

The first reason is that we have changed our nutritional habits: we rely a lot more on processed foods - pizzas, pastas, breads, potatoes, takeaways - these are a concentrated source of calories and nutrients.

We eat a lot less unprocessed foods - such as soaked grains, vegetables and fruit, seeds and nuts - than people did about 100 or 150 years ago.

Our meal times have become shorter because we don't give ourselves the luxury of sitting and enjoying our food. We end up consuming an enormous amount of calories in a very limited time.

We don't chew as much as we should; we are always in a rush. We eat the food that has been chemically enhanced, so as we put it into our mouths we are instantly aware of its taste and texture. Very few people eat hard foods that require chewing to 'unlock' their taste to the brain. Chewing also contributes to the hydration of foods. So if you don't chew, you are already dehydrated!

The other factors contributing to dehydration are stress, our overworked adrenals, air conditioning in offices, sedentary jobs, driving-everywhere lifestyles, inhaling petrol fumes, generally breathing bad air and so on.

As a rule, we do not give ourselves time to chill and slow down, do not exercise enough or, on the contrary, exercise excessively.

Dehydration is also caused by drinking sweet and fizzy drinks instead of water, drinking vast amounts of alcohol on a regular basis rather than on special occasions, regularly rather than occasionally eating substantial amounts of animal proteins.

In the meantime, our bodies need to have water all the time. We can't function without water! So, after the body has used up all the liquid it could get out of the food we have eaten, and after it has re-used the liquid stored in the digestive system, if it is still short of water, it will start searching for additional sources just to maintain its essential functions.

Water re-absorption from the bowel

There are only two storage media in the body where water is not mission-critical: fat and the stools. In order to obtain water from fat, the body needs to be involved in physical exercise over a period of time, so that the fat-burning process can release some water. It is a complicated way of "manufacturing" water in the body.

Retrieving liquid from the stools is a lot less complicated. As the large intestine receives the digested wet wastes from the small intestine to convert them further into stools, the mechanism for stool compression is already in place. About 70% of the water received from the small intestine is re-absorbed, leaving some water in the faeces for a smooth evacuation.

It also means that if we are chronically short of water, the body will obviously go to the bowel and ask for a top-up. As a result we get dry, difficult-to-pass, goat-pellet-type stools.

This applies especially to people who don't regularly eat

beans and pulses, natural grains, vegetables and fruits. The bowels of these people don't get much fibre, which helps bulk up the wastes, and consequently retain the water in the stools and stay hydrated.

Dehydration and colonics

It is not unusual to observe during a client's first colonic irrigation that no significant wastes are coming out in the first 10, 20 or even sometimes 30 minutes of the treatment! All the symptoms of the body trying to get rid of the wastes are present - the cramping, the discomfort, the urge to release - but the wastes are not coming out... guess what? The thirsty bowel is drinking water.

The poor neglected gut has been so dehydrated that it is very grateful for the unexpected supply. It is also absorbing the water into the wastes, making the wastes heavier and moister, so that eventually they will become bulky and wet enough to go through the evacuation channels.

DEHYDRATION . . . . .

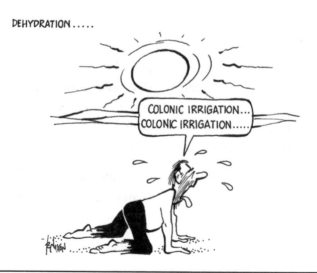

So, if that happens to you during a treatment, you know what you haven't been doing - you haven't been drinking enough water! You will eventually expel - everyone does - although it might not be a very comfortable treatment. However, you should feel much better, lighter and cleaner afterwards.

Sometimes dehydration is so severe that colon hydrotherapists do not manage to obtain a satisfying release during the first treatment. You should then continue drinking water and taking your supplements, especially the probiotic bacteria that you should be recommended. Also, increase the proportion of fresh roughage in your diet and you will see a few days after the colonic how your body starts to respond.

Again, in a situation of severe dehydration, we would recommend that you have a couple of treatments in close succession, watch the symptoms and see the difference in your body's reaction during your second treatment, and how much smoother and more comfortable the treatment becomes. It might not be perfect, but it certainly won't be as uncomfortable as the first treatment.

Came for my first colonic in early January and my bowel was so dehydrated that it took 30 minutes for it to stop having a drink. All of the water was getting soaked up before it started to clean! I felt much better afterwards and for three days finished getting rid of my de-hydrated matter.

Thanks to your wonderful advice I have completely changed my life and now have no nicotine replacement therapies or cigarettes, drink lots of water and eat a much better diet. I feel like a new woman. Now for the weight loss - had my second colonic today and it was much better and I now have lots more excellent advice to work on my figure! Thank you all very, very much!

Repair the gut wall

Repairing the gut wall is a very important task. The bowel wall has to protect our sterile internal organs, such as the liver, spleen, blood etc., from undesirable bacteria that could harm them. At the same time, it also needs to supply the same organs with nutrients, vitamins and water. Basically, it has to be both permeable and sealed.

Our skin has the same challenge. Skin is another important channel of both protection and elimination. The difference is that we can scrub the skin, rub lotions and potions into it, wash under a shower, swim in the sea, and lie in the sun. We can protect the skin against environmental damage, and generally it appears that we have a lot more control over our skin than over our gut. That is where the difficulty lies.

Four layers of the gut wall

The gut wall consists of four layers, which, for visual effect, I would like to describe as four lanes.

The first layer, mucosa, is the inside lane. It acts as a lubricant and protects the blood and other organs from gut bacteria.

The middle lane is called submucosa. It is made up of connective tissue that contains blood vessels, nerves and lymphatic vessels. It operates as an immunity barrier between the sealed eliminative system (the body's sewer) and the rest of the body. This is also where the nutrients from the large intestine are absorbed into the blood stream.

The outside lane consists of the bowel muscles that are responsible for peristaltic movement - the vertical and

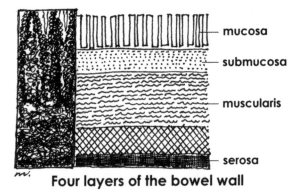

Four layers of the bowel wall

horizontal contractions that propel the faeces towards the exit.

And finally, the hard shoulder - connective tissue called serosa, which gives the gut its strength and suspends it in the chest and in the abdominal cavity. This is where the gut, in its turn, supports and massages the other internal organs.

Mucosa

There are around 200 to 500 different species of bacteria in the gut. These bacteria reside in the mucosa, weigh collectively about 1 kilogram (1 kg) and have many uses, but only inside the bowel. If they migrate to other parts of the body they can do a lot of damage. Their home is on the gut wall, and that's where they should stay.

Another important role the mucosa plays is that of protecting the rest of the body from powerful digestive enzymes produced by these bacterial colonies. These enzymes are strong enough to speed up the breakdown of indigestible fibre, called cellulose, which the rest of the body can't utilize and which mops up toxic wastes throughout the digestive system. Fermented cellulose is a foundation of a healthy elimination, so the powerful bacterial enzymes have a very important role.

Submucosa

Occasionally these strong enzymes move into the middle lane (submucosa). When they do, they can start digesting cells in that layer, in the process called autodigestion. This creates a security breach in the bowel wall, allowing toxins to escape into the blood stream and pollute the blood. This process may cause leaky gut syndrome.

Submucosa is a perennial battlefield. When undesirable bacteria penetrate the first layer of the bowel wall into the submucosal layer, the gut lymphatic system is the first line of defence. Healthy lymphatics will destroy the potential pathogens.

In a healthy body, this amazing self-regulating system works really well, but if a person is intolerant of certain foods, such as wheat, the large molecules of gluten irritate the gut wall, causing overproduction of mucus, and diarrhoea. Diarrhoea upsets the bacterial balance in the bowel, pathogens may proliferate, and breaches of mucosal security become inevitable.

Muscularis and serosa

Constipation puts excessive pressure on the connective tissue (serosa) and stretches it excessively, weakening the gut wall.

Laxatives, such as senna, and allergy triggers overexcite nerve endings in the middle lane, causing excessive peristaltic contraction in the bowel muscle and reduced absorption from the mucosa, as the immune system, alerted by the nerve endings, goes into overkill mode.

Antibiotics are equal-opportunity killers. They wipe out gut bacteria, damage the mucosal layer and increase gut permeability. The most common collateral damage caused by taking antibiotics is dysbiosis and yeast overgrowth.

One of the effects of overgrowth of the yeast *Candida albicans* is the absorption of alcohol directly into the blood stream, which weakens the immune system in the submucosa.

The colonic process

As you can see, there are many ways in which the integrity of the bowel wall can be compromised.

During colonic irrigation treatments, the mechanical action of the large amounts of clean water that are introduced into the gut dislodges any faecal matter that has dried up on the mucosal layer and is causing reduced lubrication in the bowel.

Removing wastes helps the bowel muscle to restore healthy horizontal and vertical mobility and promotes better

REPAIR THE GUT WALL.....

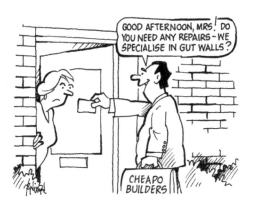

peristaltic contractions; this, in its turn, reduces pressure on the connective tissue and helps better positioning of the internal organs.

Dislodging the allergy triggers and removing them mechanically helps produce clean, healing mucus and helps repair the damaged mucosal layer. This, in its turn, ensures better absorption of nutrients and destruction of pathogens in the submucosa.

Courses of colonic irrigation treatments taken over time by habitually constipated clients have been known to rectify prolapses of the transversal colon, thus reducing the pressure on the small intestine, the uterus, the bladder and the spine. To achieve this result, the colonic treatments must be combined with a high-fibre diet, hydration, correct exercise and supplementation.

This was my fourth visit to you. I can honestly say I have gone through a life-changing experience. I have suffered with constipation all my life (now in my 50s) having relied on laxatives a lot. I have tried every sort of therapy, some helpful, some not - always ending up back where I started. I had lost hope.

The colonics have made me feel very good and the combination of the colonic and the advice on diet and exercise has all worked very effectively. I feel normal (actually better than normal) and have lost lots of bloat from my tummy area. My eyes are sparkling and I have lots more energy. What more can I ask for? Thank you!

After many years of being constipated and very miserable. I had my first colonic seven weeks ago - it was a great relief! Doctors told me I would always suffer from constipation, still nothing was done about it when it caused acute appendicitis and I was hospitalized for a week with a month off work. It has been a godsend, someone recommending colonics.

It has changed my life and improved my health 100%. Now with regular colonics and healthy eating together I feel lighter, healthier, happier and more energetic than ever before. Thank you so much, if only I knew about you years ago!

Replace digestants and rebalance the bowel flora

You have no doubt heard about the 'good bacteria' and 'bad bacteria' that live in the bowel. This can sometimes create a wrong impression: many people believe that the gut is some kind of a battleground between Good and Evil. What it really means, though, is that some bacteria play a negative role while others play a positive role in the processes of absorption and elimination that take place in the bowel.

The bowel's ecosystem

Generally, the bowel is a host to numerous colonies of bacteria - there are between 200 and 500 species in total - and each colony plays an important part in absorption, vitamin and enzyme production, stools formation and elimination.

To get a better idea of the role of bacteria, we should remember that some of them are designed to mop up our carbohydrate waste and fibre, and some of them are designed to deal with the protein waste that we have in our bowels. The correct balance between these organisms will determine how successful and comfortable our bowel movements are. Some of these organisms are weaker, and some of them are stronger. Historically, some of them in the course of human development, have played a more important role; some of them are on standby and only come into their own at times of crisis, such as in food poisoning or when there are hormonal changes.

Everyone is unique, and every nation's bowel bacterial make-up tends to be influenced, to an extent, by dietary traditions formed over centuries. Northern Europeans, who for centuries have had a high proportion of muscle and organ meat, milk and milk products in their diets, are different in their bacterial make-up from South Americans, who eat mainly grains and root vegetables, or Eskimos, who eat a lot of fish or Mongols who don't eat vegetables at all!

The basics of good stools

RESPECT FOR YOUR INTERNAL FLORA.....

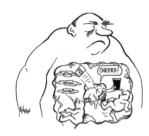

Nevertheless, there are commonalities amongst all people. One of the things that everyone has in common is that their stools consist of dead blood cells, stomach and intestinal cells, fibre and indigestible wastes. Also everyone's stools need to be fermented in order to be eliminated.

The 'backbone' of good stools is fermented fibre. Fibre, both soluble and insoluble, is a carbohydrate, so everyone needs plenty of bacteria that are able to assist in the fermentation of carbohydrate wastes.

If you do not eat enough grains, pulses, fruit or vegetables containing good, strong fibre, in all likelihood you will not have enough bacteria in your bowel to be able to process fibre into good quality stools, because there is no call for these bacteria to be present.

If you also eat processed foods or a diet high in proteins, it is more likely that you will have bacteria that facilitate the putrefaction of proteins. In small quantities, these bacteria would do absolutely no harm, but if you have an imbalanced diet you will also have an imbalanced bacterial make-up.

Colonic irrigation and gut bacteria

It is said sometimes that colonic irrigation washes out good bacteria.

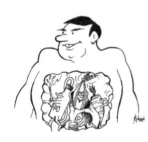

RESPECT FOR YOUR INTERNAL FLORA...

Logically, if your bowel were colonized with a balanced mix of beneficial bacteria that created good-quality stools (that is the majority of fibre-fermenting bacteria, and a small number of bacteria that speed up the protein putrefaction process), they would be removed in equal ratios during the colonic treatment.

If after the colonic treatment you follow a diet that is rich in natural yoghurt, fresh fruit and vegetables and sprouted grains, this would encourage the preservation and proliferation of beneficial bacteria.

If you feel the need for your colonic treatment because you are experiencing discomfort in your bowel, then probably one of the main reasons for this discomfort is the overproduction of putrefying bacteria and the shortage of fibre-fermenting bacteria.

In this case, a colonic treatment would help restore the equilibrium of bacteria by giving you an opportunity to restart good nutrition and promote the growth of fibre-fermenting bacteria.

After the colonic treatment, your therapist may recommend taking a probiotic supplement and live yoghurts.

Probiotic supplements and live yoghurts help maintain an acidic environment in the large intestine, which encourages the growth of the bacteria that digest carbohydrates and fibre, and that help in their fermentation and in the creation of good, soft stools, as well as in the retention of moisture in the stools. This would also give stool-forming bacteria a good start.

So, in general, if you use colon hydrotherapy as a cleansing and educational tool at regular intervals, this will enable you to give a boost to your elimination system every time and help the bowel to rebalance its bacteria.

Colon hydrotherapy can help kick-start the habit of good nutrition and make you more conscious of the need to be more connected to your body.

After suffering severe constipation for many years, I decided to have a colonic irrigation. After 3 treatments and a change in eating habits, and supplements, the results have been dramatic. I would recommend it for anyone with similar problems. It is not just a one-off treatment, regular maintenance is also key and the advice and treatment you receive are brilliant.

Restore the bowel function

Restoration of bowel function and bowel regularity is one of the most important goals of colon hydrotherapy treatments.

Very often those who embark on a good diet and lifestyle without a bowel cleanse find it very difficult to notice any obvious changes in their wellbeing and in the activity of their bowel.

There might be quite a few reasons for this, but one of the most obvious reasons is that they have still got too much old faecal matter in their bowels. So whatever they do, their bowels are not working at 100% efficiency - the mucosa can't self-lubricate and the gut muscles can't contract and relax properly because the gut is still too full.

The gut gets a workout

Removing the faecal matter enables the bowel muscle to work better. This, in turn, will help with the absorption of nutrients and the production of the B and K vitamins that the bowel requires for its optimal functioning.

As better-fermented, heavier and moister stools are created, they give a better workout to the bowel muscle. A properly exercised muscle, in its turn, is more aware of the signals sent by the nerve endings, and delivers the stools through the rectum and the anal canal for regular elimination.

As you empty more fully, the muscle remains in good shape, no plaque develops on the bowel walls, and the effective digestion, absorption, assimilation and elimination continue.

We also need to remember that one of the functions of the

bowel that is often taken for granted is the support and massage it provides to other internal organs in the thoracic and the abdominal cavities.

The regular peristaltic action massages the stomach, the spleen and the liver above the transverse colon, and provides support and a frame to the small intestine and the organs of the abdominal cavity. An oversized gut stifles the organs rather than supporting them.

A prolapsed transverse colon would put the whole of the abdominal cavity under pressure, as well as the kidneys and the abdomen, which rely on the transverse colon for support.

Getting rid of the excess baggage that constipated people often carry around in their bowels has been known to relieve back and chest pain, help with the constant urge to urinate by reducing the pressure on the bladder, stop heavy bleeding during periods, and increase the chances of pregnancy.

Thank you for another colonic. I cannot believe how much healthier I feel and look now. Having suffered ongoing illnesses through work stress, I damaged my body with the continuous antibiotics prescribed, I finally feel myself again. Actually I feel a lot better if I'm honest!

I've changed my diet, which is significant when I consider what I ate before (serious sugar and chocoholic, plus a ready made meal queen!). It made me moody in the first week, but I got over myself. Now I enjoy a 'beauty breakfast' and don't crave the bad stuff. The best bit for me is that I have always had skin problems, on my arms and back; an unusual situation that no dermatologists could solve.

After a decade of trying everything under the sun, my skin is clear and glowing, just one month after following Galina's advice. Incredible! I now get comments on how my eyes and skin are twinkling and glowing. How nice! I feel healthy enough to get back into the world of work - but this time I will do it right; fewer hours and no more ready meals. Thank you all.

Rebuild the brain-gut connection

The brain-gut connection is something everyone is aware of, albeit not consciously: every time we need to make an important phone call, or make a decision that involves risk, we have a feeling of 'butterflies in the stomach'.

The expression 'gut feeling' is used to describe a premonition that exists on the visceral level and is not supported by any facts that the head could rely on to make a decision. Shocking news may leave us doubled up with abdominal pain or gasping for breath. Diarrhoea on the night before an important exam is quite common.

This is all the part of 'fight or flight' mechanism that regulates our response to danger. We are programmed to respond like this.

Our gut is also programmed to tell us when we are hungry, when we have had enough food and when we need to open our bowels to eliminate the wastes.

About 95% of the available serotonin, the neurotransmitter better known as the mood regulator, is stored in the gut. The bowel and the head constantly exchange messages, although in most people this is a one-way street: apparently, 9 out of 10 messages are sent upwards. So in a way, our gut determines our mood.

That is why our bowel is often called 'the second brain'.

The Second Brain

THE BOWEL IS OUR
SECOND BRAIN.....

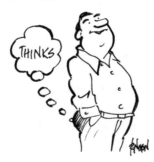

The second brain, or the enteric nervous system, i.e. the nervous system that operates the digestive system, can and should work independently from the head.

Once we have swallowed a portion of food, the next time we will have any conscious control over it is when we open our bowel. The whole process of transformation of food into nutrients, and of nutrients into our cells, happens virtually without involving our 'head brain'.

Listening to your body

Precisely because of this, 'listening to your body' makes so much sense. It should be pretty straightforward: chew your food, wait for the signs of satiety, stop eating, and let the body digest, absorb and discard; listen to your body again, open your bowel and eliminate.

We know what happens instead: we eat not only for hunger, but often for pleasure, consolation or greed; we don't open our bowels when they ask us to, because we think it's the wrong place or the wrong time; we ignore the signs of satiety and eat up everything in sight; we do not chew; we do not hydrate ourselves and so on.

So we should not be surprised when the gut sends upwards plenty of messages saying that it is bloated, irritated, constipated, spastic and full of indigestible materials that even bacteria refuse to deal with!

Serotonin overflows, causing diarrhoea, which in turn shuts off the serotonin receptors in the gut, causing constipation. This is how the IBS cycle works, creating spasms and irritation of the bowel wall.

As a result, the head brain receives a lot of unhappy messages.

Rebuilding fundamental links

Colonic irrigation helps restore the healthy brain-gut connection in several ways.

When the water flow causes the bowel to evacuate the wastes, it rebuilds the fundamental link that is compromised in so many people - the urge to open the bowel followed by immediate evacuation. Both the head and the gut brains remember it; it feels natural, it feels good and it feels right. Colonics begin to re-establish this very important neural pathway.

This basic reflex is part of the programming that we are born with. It should be our default mode, and many people who follow the post-colonic dietary recommendations and hydrate themselves notice after the first couple of colonics that they 'know better' when to go, and that they are much more aware of the need to give themselves time to evacuate wastes.

Relieving bowel spasms

A lot of the unhappiness and moodiness of people who suffer from the symptoms of irritable bowel is caused by the bowel going into spasm day after day, virtually after every meal. This is often caused by the bacterial imbalance, mucosal wall irritation and the presence of allergy triggers.

Colonics executed with very warm water help relieve the bowel spasm by mechanically relaxing the muscle layer of the bowel. Relaxation of the muscles gives a positive message to the nerves that regulate serotonin production. As a temporary measure, this often helps reduce considerably the symptoms of IBS, giving the body and mind a welcome break from its niggling symptoms.

This, in combination with proper chewing, small, warm meals and more specific dietary measures, brings relief from IBS much faster than dietary measures alone.

Mechanical removal of allergy triggers from the bowel helps calm down the inflamed nerve endings, regulating the serotonin production and relieving the symptoms of chronic diarrhoea.

Resolving negativity

Colon hydrotherapy also helps many people who 'bottle up' their emotions to start the process of emotional clearout. Emotions are, on a very basic level, electric charges. Storing a lot of negativity in the gut does not do much good to its balance.

Getting rid of this negativity may cause emotional upset in some people.

If this is what happens to you, it can only mean one thing - you need 'closure'. You have to deal with stored-up issues that are trying to escape. Go with the flow: trust your gut.

In many more people, whose 'negative charge' was not excessive, the clearout causes a great feeling of the 'incredible lightness of being' at every level: physical, emotional, intellectual and spiritual.

That is why quite a few of creative people have colonics to get rid of writer's block and to obtain a surge of fresh adrenalin.

The Bottom Line

Basically, if the only newsflash you get from your rear end is the daily need to open your bowels, your digestive system must be working well. Once you start getting more frequent progress reports, and they don't 'feel right', go with your gut feeling and give the bowel a good clearout!

 I'm back. Just had my second colonic with Galina. I feel great! After my last one I slightly changed my diet as per your expert advice and started drinking lots more water, and guess what?? NOT CONSTIPATED ANY MORE! Thank you very much for the advice. The whole experience for me has been fantastic - I will definitely come again. Now to try some 'dry skin brushing!'

Re-educate the owner of the bowel

I was seriously tempted to call this book 'The Bowel Owner's Manual', because that is exactly what it is!

This is the one subject about which I feel very evangelical and for which my passion for helping people becomes almost an obsession - colonics can change people's lives, but only if they are ready for the change.

For many people, opting for colonic irrigation is a great step towards taking control of their own health. The first step is never easy. We all feel very proprietary about 'down there', and allowing a foreign mechanical device to enter our very private space requires courage and determination.

Once everything is in place and the treatment starts, you feel like you are on a personal growth rollercoaster ride.

The visual impact

If you can see the wastes, the treatment has an amazing visual impact.

Watching the wastes being washed away makes you feel good and clean; it is, in a way, like being in a confession booth: saying where you have gone wrong to a total stranger behind the wall somehow helps you to let go and often brings a long-awaited closure.

Many people, seeing how much waste their bodies are able to store, are awed. They decide, there and then, to change their diet for the better, to exercise more and never again to let their body amass so much rubbish.

I have seen people undergo a great transformation in a heartbeat: all the things they have read about the need to exercise their bodies, about eating fresh vegetables and fruit, chewing food and drinking water suddenly come together in a great visual splash.

Emotional release

The emotional release during colonics can be quite amazing. Often, for those who find it difficult to let go, nothing happens at the start of the treatment. Then - just one word from the therapist, one question, one look - will open a flood gate, and tears and wastes leave the body together, creating a space for new, positive emotions in the soul and for better absorption and assimilation in the body.

WE DO NOT HAVE ANY RESERVATIONS ABOUT CLEANING OUR TEETH......

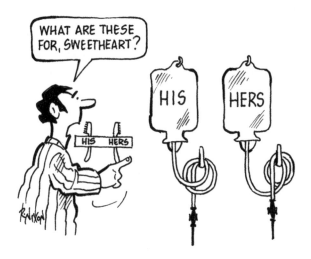

Your curiosity about how your body works is aroused, you feel the cathartic power of self-cleansing and, in a way, life will never be the same again!

Also, with each treatment you will learn more and more about your body. Don't be afraid of asking your therapist questions, and of finding out how you can use colonics to promote your health, longevity and wellbeing.

Often, after a good colonic, people are determined to live a much healthier lifestyle.

Just keep going!

As time goes on, most of us tend to lower our standards little by little. We think we can get away with more - familiarity breeds contempt, as they say. We allow ourselves more nutritional luxuries. We exercise less. We eat more. We forget about lymph cleansing, we don't go for our regular massages and all of a sudden one day we notice that we've become sluggish again.

This is not surprising. Looking after your bowel is hard work and in modern life there are many other things competing for your time and attention.

Once you have found that you have become a little bit too sluggish, book yourself in for another treatment and start the self-improvement curve again. What you need to do is to find your comfort zone, and normally three to four colonic treatments a year will give you a good overall result.

 I have received 2 colonics at Wellbeing Now and the experiences after the colonics have changed my eating habits for life and overall stress management. I am quite a private person so when people comment on how well I look, I simply thank them - and do not pass comment. Now, I comment and say this treatment is simple, proven and will definitely make a difference. Today I have received my third colonic and again it was amazing. Thank you, I can't praise you all enough.

Thanks! I haven't felt so good in ages. The colonic was comfortable and your advice was very helpful I would recommend this to anyone; it just makes you think about what damage we are doing to ourselves!

When I first came here three weeks ago for my first colonic, I was a 6'2', 19 and a half stone walking heart attack. It was time to make some changes. The treatment was the start of some major changes in lifestyle. I've lost over a stone in the three weeks since and I suspect a whole lot more will follow. Thank you for the kick-start I so desperately needed.

Colon hydrotherapy and you

If you want to get the best value out of your treatments, there are certain things you need to know.

No two people are the same; everyone is unique. It is important to understand your own personal reasons for opting to have colon hydrotherapy treatments and what you personally want to get out of these procedures.

The following are the potential benefits, so if you want to use this book as your road map, you can tick the boxes that could be important for you:

If you are new to colonics, there may be only two or three things that you would wish to gain, here and now. As your relation with your body deepens, there will be other things - probably more physical, probably more spiritual or emotional - that colon hydrotherapy may help you achieve.

Put a date next to your answers, and as you revisit this section of the book from time to time, you will be able to see how your priorities have evolved.

Additional benefits

The table overleaf covers most, but by far not all the benefits of having colon hydrotherapy treatments. Colonics may help resolve more specialist problems, related to sex drive, infertility and other hormonal imbalances. A good general practitioner who uses both mainstream and alternative medicine would be able to advise you further. Homeopathy and herbalism in combination with colonics and bodywork are also very effective.

WHAT CAN BE GAINED FROM COLONIC IRRIGATION	Date								
Flushing the large intestine, removing wastes from your gut									
Using the treatment as prevention against degenerative diseases									
Helping with IBS, feeling of bloatedness, constipation or bouts of diarrhoea									
Helping with the strengthening of the immune system									
Contributing to liver, blood and kidney cleansing									
Helping to clear up the skin and symptoms of acne, and to remove dark bags under the eyes									
Increasing energy level, stamina; reducing the need for long sleeps									
Exercising your bowel muscle, helping it to become more active in eliminating toxins									
Restoring the correct balance of beneficial bacteria in your gut									

Helping to manage yeast overgrowth, signs of gut dysbiosis or Candida							
Helping with weight loss and long-term weight management							
Helping to manage food, alcohol and cigarette cravings							
Helping with the release of emotional wastes stored in the large bowel							
Helping to manage intolerances, such as gluten, processed wheat etc.							
As a visual reinforcement of the need to eat healthily and hydrate your body							
Contributing to your deeper understanding about your own body							
Reinforcing your desire for self-improvement and healthy living							
As a component of your personal growth and development programme							

Seven months ago my problems began. Every single day my tummy would bloat massively and it lasted about 4 to 6 hours, causing discomfort and backache. The doctor said it was due to wind and acid and prescribed numerous lotions and potions. Nothing worked.

I then took matters into my own hands and found a nutritionist. Six days into my new eating habits all was going well until I became constipated. A week later, back to the doctor. Now I was prescribed laxatives - in all 9 different ones.... Nothing worked and X-rays and ultrasounds confirmed an impacted colon. 56 days later, I still had not been to the loo.

I felt and looked awful and on the point of death. The doctor and hospital said there was nothing more they could do except bowel surgery to remove the impaction. Great. I was surely going to die now from peritonitis.

Once again I took matters into my own hands and booked a colonic. I was very nervous but needn't have been. Everyone at Wellbeing Now is friendly, helpful and hell bent on improving your quality of life. 5 weeks after my colonic, I'm back again with my husband this time. He was so amazed at the changes in me, he too needed no persuading.

The cause of all my problems... TOO MANY ANTIBIOTICS, which had completely destroyed the good bugs in my gut, leaving it unable to function at all. Thank you to the doctors!!! Its cost me a great deal of money for prescription just to make me ill! Today I am a new person, ready to live life again. Thank you so much for your help and care. This was the best thing I have ever done in my life.

Main types of colonic equipment

What you need to know when deciding what equipment to use

There are two main types of colon hydrotherapy systems used in professional practices.

The first type is usually described as 'an open system'.

In an open system, that is based on the use of cool and warm water flush with gravity, there is one thin rectal tube that allows water into the rectum, while the waste matter is released directly from the rectum into an opening in a special colonic chair and straight into a waste tube.

This type of equipment is popular mainly in the USA and Australia but has yet to become established in the professional colon hydrotherapy market in the UK.

The other system is 'a closed system' originally designed by Dr. Robert A. Wood which also combines cool and warm water flush with the use of gravity. Dr. Wood began his career in Australia, his native land, in 1914. As his research into human health and disease progressed, he found that this method of bowel cleansing was the most effective and safe way to clean the entire large intestine.

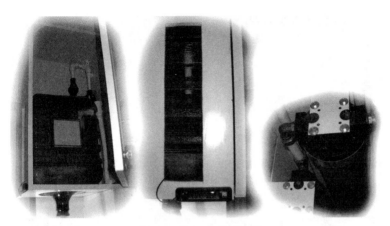

Modern gravity colon hydrotherapy unit, showing the water tank and the filters

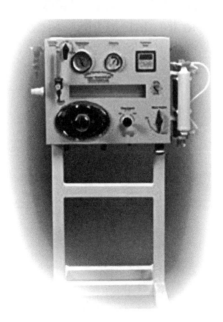

Modern colon therapy pressure device

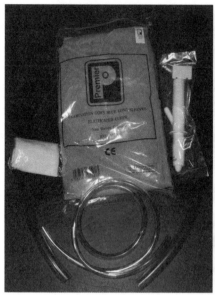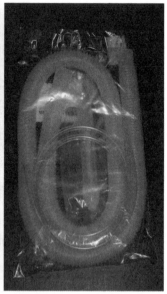

Disposable treatment kits - recommended

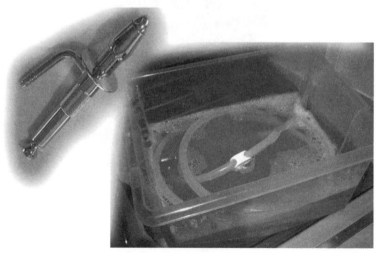

**Reusable speculum and pipe sterilization system
- not recommended**

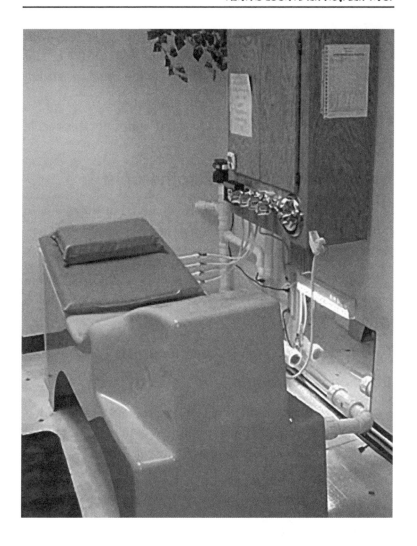

The open colon hydrotherapy system

A variation of the closed system is a pressure system, with which the treatment is performed using a colonic device and pressure, rather than gravity. Colonic devices are also quickly gaining popularity in the UK.

All colonic equipment can be used with fully disposable kits.

Finding your colon hydrotherapist

Usually you brush your teeth yourself, but from time to time you need the assistance of a dental hygienist who gives them a good spring cleaning.

In the same way, most healthy people would benefit from having their gut periodically groomed by a professional colon hydrotherapist.

Two types of colon hydrotherapists

Traditional approach

As with any therapy, establishing a contact and an understanding with your therapist would be extremely important when you embark on colon hydrotherapy treatments.

There are two approaches to colon hydrotherapy and two types of colon hydrotherapists.

The first approach is to consider colon hydrotherapy to be an extremely powerful treatment that can bring changes to your digestion and elimination without much effort on your part. Supporters of this approach usually advocate having an initial series of six or twelve colonic treatments booked closely together, in a space of weeks or months. Dietary advice is generally not individualized, and there is not much emphasis

BRIEF GUIDE TO CHOOSING THE COLONIC EQUIPMENT

It is very important to choose the equipment that meets your needs fully.

Remember that a professional therapist will give a satisfying treatment with any equipment (please see below how to choose your therapist).

Manually operated Woods Gravity System: This is the original system, and most colonic therapists practicing in the UK have been trained to perform the treatment using this system. It requires therapist's presence and full involvement during the whole procedure. The system is very adjustable and the therapist can vary the pressure of the flow and the temperature of the water depending on the client's reaction. Fully disposable kits can be used. Depending on the type of outlet pipes used with kits, the client may be able to see the wastes that come out.

Advantages: Adjusts extremely well to diverse needs of clients. Easy to keep clean if disposables are used. You will be able to gain knowledge by working with the therapist during the treatment.

Disadvantages: Many traditional therapists still use non-disposable equipment.

The Open System: This is a 'Plug and Play' system. The treatment is performed using a special colonic chair. A small speculum, no wider than a pencil, is inserted into the rectum by the client gently wriggling onto the speculum. Often the therapist explains how to regulate the water temperature and leaves the client to self-administer the treatment.

Advantages: Private and discreet. Gives a good wash.

Disadvantages: You may not gain much knowledge. If you don't know what you are doing, you may feel insecure at the start. Hygiene is of utmost importance due to a large contact area with the human body.

Mechanically Operated System: Colonic devices warm their own water. They work on feedback pressure from the client's bowels, and the process of filling up the client with water and releasing it is more automated than using either an open or a closed gravity system. Therefore the treatment may feel like less "hands-on". The client should always be able to see the wastes. The therapist is present throughout the treatment (check it though).

Advantages: The client should always be able to see the wastes. Disposable kits are used. The equipment is easy to clean and filters its own water.

Disadvantages: Sometimes it may be less comfortable than the other two systems because the machine is more in control, and the machine cannot know what you are feeling. Some devices do not have a mechanical break required by the UK Water Board.

Questions to ask: What system do you use? Is the therapist going to be present throughout the procedure? How long is the water treatment procedure? (Should be around 45 to 60 minutes). What parts of your kit are disposable? Are the inlet and the outlet pipes disposable? Will I be able to see the wastes?

on exercise or supplementation.

This approach certainly has its merits, because it subjects the body to shock therapy, and the body has to mobilize all its systems, all its defences and all its resources to start functioning better.

As you follow the course of the treatment and deep cleansing is introduced to the colon, promoting the elimination of waste, your blood gets cleaner and your kidneys and liver are detoxified. This normally leads to important positive changes.

Many traditionally trained colon hydrotherapists pursue this approach. This approach is widely propagated in the information circulated by major colon hydrotherapy organizations etc.

The advantage of this approach for you, as a client or a patient, is that it is easy. All you need is to turn up and pay the money. Visits to the colon hydrotherapists would be akin to visits to your doctor. You come in, the doctor gives you a pill, you take the pill, and that effects the changes you wish to achieve (or sometimes it does not).

Naturopathic approach

The second approach is what could be described as a naturopathic approach. Naturopaths believe that great changes can be achieved in a person's health by involving the person's consciousness, focus and intellect. They believe in educating their clients. Bernard Jensen, one of the most outstanding naturopaths and lateral thinkers the 20th century was advocating this approach when talking about colon hydrotherapy.

In his classic essay, *'Tissue Cleansing through Bowel Management'*, he wrote that colonics vary greatly in their effects due largely to the expertise of the colonic therapist or technician. He felt that in some respects colon hydrotherapy was taking advantage of people by making them believe that long and costly treatments were necessary.

Jensen was convinced that those practitioners who administered colon hydrotherapy properly were offering a useful service to the public, with the addition of sound dietary counselling and knowledge so as to eventually overcome the need for the treatment itself.

Bernard Jensen said: *'Without this knowledge, the colonic recipient is merely digging holes and filling them again - a net zero toward building a better health quality. Many professionals giving colonics today are getting successful but temporary results.*

CONSTIPATION.....

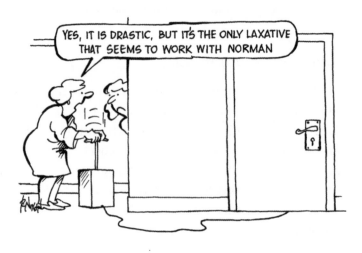

YES, IT IS DRASTIC, BUT IT'S THE ONLY LAXATIVE THAT SEEMS TO WORK WITH NORMAN

The reason for this is that just getting rid of the toxic waste in the bowel is not the complete answer, although it is the first step along the correct path. Unless proper exercise, diet and right living are practiced, good and lasting results will not be achieved. We must be interested in making bowel tissue changes'. (Published by Bernard Jensen D.C, Ph.D 1981, p. 90).

Naturopathic colon hydrotherapists believe that the treatments itself, although crucially important, is only the start of the cleansing process. A naturopathic consultant would probably encourage you to have two or three treatments initially, in the first couple of months.

You will also need to do some work between treatments: focus on your water intake, on your chewing, on your physical activity and emotional life, on making step-by-step changes in your diet, and often on taking supplements that will encourage the restoration of the digestive processes that have caused your colonic disturbances in the first place.

A typical session with a naturopathic colon hydrotherapist would involve filling in a questionnaire, which focuses on the reasons why you wish to have a colonic treatment, as well as on your general wellbeing. In the process of the treatment, a naturopathic consultant would certainly talk to you a lot.

The consultant might not even ask you what you eat; but may talk about your family and about your personal life, in hope of finding a trigger that caused the imbalance that has brought you for treatment. The therapist would want to focus on the one thing, the main link, that is affecting your wellbeing, and try to help you reconnect this missing link.

Aftercare

Traditional colon hydrotherapists focus mainly on the bowel, while naturopathic hydrotherapists look at the bowel as an integral part of the whole person.

Therefore after the end of the treatment, traditional colon hydrotherapists and naturopathic colon hydrotherapists would prescribe slightly different regimens for your wellbeing.

Taking, for example, constipation, which is one of the main reasons people have the colonic sessions: traditional colon hydrotherapists may recommend supplements that have a laxative effect on the bowel, sometimes with the added benefit of liver cleansing. They often recommend a series of at least six treatments.

Naturopathic colon hydrotherapists would probably focus on probiotics that encourage the survival of beneficial bacteria in your bowel. They would advise you on supplements that promote general digestive and emotional health, such as glutamine, soya lecithin, MSM, the B complex, magnesium etc.

They might encourage you to make fresh vegetable juice, to use more bitter herbs, to breathe differently, to do some yoga, to use lymphatic exercise such as rebounding, to dry skin brush, and generally to invoke the body's own healing forces to help your elimination system to work more actively.

Naturopathic colon hydrotherapists are often reluctant to use laxative substances, and would only resort to them as a short-term measure. Typically they would wait for between two and eight weeks before repeating your treatment, and at the second or third treatment they would encourage you to establish your own pattern of therapeutic colonic maintenance.

Most people have three or four treatments a year, or slightly more, as they grow older.

Sometimes more treatments can be beneficial at the start, if someone suffers from a serious condition or disease. Under these circumstances, working in close contact with a naturopathically minded doctor would certainly be recommended

Various ways of conducting a treatment

Therapists are also different in the way they conduct colon hydrotherapy treatments. Some are more hands-on, using massage, reflexology, breathing therapy, infrared light or ultrasound waves to relax you and let you enjoy the benefit of the therapeutic touch, while at the same time encouraging the bowel to release the waste.

Other therapists, especially those who work with open system equipment or automated colonic devices, which are generally less dependent on the therapist's input, tend to conduct the treatment at arm's length. Sometimes they may even leave you on your own, although the guidelines of all major colonic organizations expressly disapprove of this practice.

How important is therapists' education and colonic training?

To understand the different pathways that can be taken to become a colon hydrotherapist, we need to look back at the period between the middle of the 1960s and the second half of the 1990s.

Before the 1960s colon hydrotherapy was widely used as part of spa and sanatoria regimen, as well as being performed in doctors' surgeries. Colon hydrotherapy devices - 'machines' - were quite common, both in Europe and in the USA.

With further development of the pharmaceutical industry, people have started to rely on more pills for the management of their numerous ailments.

Pills are certainly cheaper to administer, and the logistics of administering a pill are considerably more straightforward than the logistics of administering colon hydrotherapy treatments. It is certainly easier to dispense a supply of laxatives to a client than to bring that person into a surgery for colon hydrotherapy treatment by a doctor or a nurse.

From the 1960s colon hydrotherapy started to be viewed by the medical community as an inessential practice. Those who continued to practise colon hydrotherapy were mostly former nurses, or alternative therapists, often working from their therapy rooms at home or in small alternative practices, usually obtaining their clients by recommendation and working in relative isolation from other practitioners.

There were few larger practices, medical or holistic, that offered this service to their clients, and until very recently there were only two schools in the UK that trained colon hydrotherapists.

USA training

In the USA, colon hydrotherapy remained much more popular. It was actively promoted by manufacturers of colon hydrotherapy devices, who also encouraged education and continuing professional development. One of these manufacturers even set up an association, the International Association of Colon Therapists (or I-ACT), which is now the largest association of colon hydrotherapists in the world with over 1,700 members.

Colon hydrotherapists in the USA mostly have been trained to use automated colonic devices and, for the last 30 years, have been actively encouraged to use disposable equipment.

Anyone who is passionate about colon health can be trained as a colon hydrotherapist in the USA. The I-ACT syllabus places considerable emphasis on the anatomy and physiology of the human body, on doing a large number of treatments in the course of training, and on colon and treatment hygiene.

Therapists are originally trained as hygienists, who may not be able to recommend dietary changes or supplementation. However, there is a structured path of professional growth that enables I-ACT therapists to enhance their skills.

I-ACT is also becoming more popular in the UK. There is now an I-ACT approved school in London that follows a USA system of training.

UK training

Colon hydrotherapy schools in the UK treat colonic irrigation as a postgraduate modality. They accept therapists who should already have prior knowledge of anatomy and experience of bodywork, and teach them the treatment technique and some of the related modalities. UK-trained colon therapists were traditionally trained on gravity colonic units and non-disposable equipment, but with a more hands-on approach. This situation is changing now, as colonic devices are making inroads into the British market.

Therapists who were trained in the UK were encouraged to join UK colon hydrotherapy associations; the main one now is the Association and Register of Colon Hydrotherapists (ARCH).

Association membership

Some therapists join both I-ACT and ARCH, whilst some are not members of any colonic practitioner organizations.

Membership of an association can be important, because traditionally associations purport to give some sort of assurance about the quality of one's work.

However, membership alone is not everything. I have had colonic treatments from very good non-associated practitioners. For me, a very important question to ask is what other modalities the colon therapist practises or encourages, such as naturopathy, nutrition, herbalism, hypnotherapy, aromatherapy, massage and so on.

Also it is worth inquiring when choosing your colon therapist whether the person is a member of any other professional associations, such as a nutritionists' or naturopaths' governing body, or the Federation of Holistic Therapists, Beauty Guild, etc.

Larger associations, such as the Federation of Holistic Therapists, the Beauty Guild and I-ACT, have more resources to conduct and encourage continuing professional development. They also offer more opportunities for members practising colonics and other complementary therapies to meet together and exchange views.

The personality factor

You would be reluctant to believe the advice of a dietician who has bad skin and bad breath and who is seriously over-weight and looks unhealthy. You probably wouldn't take the advice of a cardiac consultant who chain-smokes. You would hesitate to go to a dentist who has rotten, yellow teeth.

So it is equally important to see that your colon hydrotherapist actually looks healthy and radiates health, energy and a positive lifestyle. Choose someone whose example would encourage you to make positive changes in the same way as having a fit and good-looking personal trainer with good muscle definition would encourage you to exercise more.

Look for a therapist who meets your needs

Some therapists successfully use infrared heat, some use alternating hot and cold water, some use massage, some use reflexology, some use relaxation techniques, some get you to talk about something that is important to you so that you focus your attention on your own priorities.

Every therapist will find his or her own way of making the colonic release more comfortable and successful. However if you have had a treatment and the therapist did not use any supporting techniques, and you did not get a satisfactory release, it is probably worth looking for someone else and trying to find a therapist who would be likely to meet your needs in a more comprehensive way.

The importance of disposable equipment

Most colon hydrotherapists who trained in the UK did so using non-disposables. Many of them have since moved to using disposable equipment, because it is more hygienic and presents a much lesser risk of contamination.

When inquiring about disposable equipment, you should ask whether the therapist uses just a disposable speculum (a plastic tube that is inserted into your anus) or if they also use disposable inlet pipe and outlet pipes.

It is worth paying a little bit extra for a fully disposable kit, because, again, this is a safer and more hygienic approach to giving colonic treatment.

Treatment procedure and commonly asked questions

You probably wonder what to expect during your colon hydrotherapy treatment. Obviously, a lot will depend on your initial state of health and on the extent of the co-operation of your digestive system during the treatment.

If you are a healthy person with a reasonably good diet, with regular bowel movement (a satisfying release at least five or six times a week), you can expect to have a comfortable and short treatment (around 30 minutes).

While the water fills your bowels, you will probably experience a 'bizarre' sensation or cramps as the wastes and the water move towards the anus for evacuation. As the treatment progresses, a longer section of the bowel will be cleared of the residual waste and you will be able to hold the water for longer, thus encouraging it to wash out the more remote

COLON THERAPY AND YOU.....

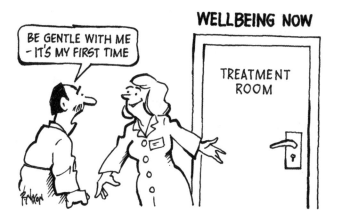

recesses of your intestines.

You should bear in mind that your large bowel is approximately the same length as your body from head to toe, and that it fits into quite a small area in your body. Therefore, you should try to encourage the water to travel up and down the curves of your bowel, and 'go inland' to the extent that it is reasonably comfortable for you, removing on the way back the wastes that have accumulated on the bowel wall.

In letting the water fill your bowel, it is useful to apply the same rule that wise people use for routine muscle stretching: on an exertion scale of 1 to 10, never push your body past the 7.5 mark.

If you feel that too much water is making you really uncomfortable, you should ask your therapist to stop filling and let the water flow out. Ask for a break if you feel you need one. Remember, this is your body after all.

The Small Print

The answers below are general - they apply to reasonably healthy people who wish to become healthier, rather than to people who are very unwell and who wish to become well.

You are generally healthy if you are able to work, rest, have a relationship or family, etc, in a word, just live a normal life. Becoming healthier means, for example, getting rid of constipation, bloatedness, bad skin, bad breath, extra pounds and diarrhoea; as well as learning more about yourself, raising your energy levels and gaining more control over your eating and relaxation habits.

You are ill if you have a condition that precludes you from living a generally healthy life, as described above.

Colonic irrigation can be, and is, successfully used to treat serious life-threatening and debilitating conditions, such as cancer, autoimmune diseases, multiple sclerosis, advanced stages of fibromyalgia, ME and many others.

You can have colonics and all related treatments - and probably should do so - if you are suffering from a serious disease. Under these circumstances, I would recommend you to contact a holistic doctor or a representative from a holistic health institution, such as the Hippocrates Institute in Florida, Paracelsus in Switzerland, Sanoviv, or The Oasis of Hope in Mexico.

These institutions specialize in the holistic management of serious and life-threatening conditions and achieve amazing results with a lot of people.

Can anyone have this treatment?

Most people can have colonics; but in certain situations colonic treatments are contraindicated or must only be under-taken only by a trained medical practitioner in a hospital setting. The list of seven major contraindications to the colonic treatment is below.

**SEVEN CONTRAINDICATIONS TO
COLONIC IRRIGATION**

1. **congestive heart failure**

2. **severe anaemia**

3. **pregnancy, especially the first trimester (medical supervision recommended afterwards)**

Inflammatory conditions in an acute form such as:

4. **diverticulitis, ulcerative colitis, Crohn's disease**

5. **severe hemorrhoids**

6. **a tumor in the rectum or large intestine**

7. **recent colorectal surgery**

What should I do before the treatment?

If this is your first colonic treatment and you want to use it as body maintenance, cleansing and an educational experi-ence, it is probably best to do nothing beforehand.

The treatment will reflect your current state of health: the extent to which your bowel is able to get rid of the faecal matter, the state of hydration of your bowel, the state of communication between your bowel and brain and, generally, your body's efficiency at eliminating wastes.

Start being healthy right now!

If you are already aware of what to expect, a good idea would be to start eating lighter, smaller meals, drinking more liquids, making fresh vegetable juices, probably exercising more, and generally grooming your body for a good elimination.

On the day of the colonics, we recommend eating light meals and not having any food for an hour and a half to two hours before the treatment. Wear comfortable clothes. This is a general rule when you have any kind of bodywork done. We also suggest that you keep the rest of the day for relaxation to enable your body to continue the cleansing process.

Is anything added to the water?

Some therapists add cleansing herbs (which promote elimination), Epsom salts, ozone and other substances to the water.

I never add anything during the first treatment, as I use colonics not only as a cleansing tool, but also as an educational tool for my clients, explaining to them what I see. I try and make the treatment visual, educational and memorable - in a good sense.

For me, the colour and the quality of the stools are really important. Some of the other things I look at are the speed of eliminations and the extent of the bowel's involvement in the cleansing process (i.e., how much the bowel contributes to the process as opposed to what is the result of the cleansing effect of the water itself).

For this reason, water is an ideal medium: with water, what you see is what you get. A client's subsequent treatments might involve using Epsom salts, probiotic solutions or herbal tinctures. However, I do rely on water alone, most of the time.

Do I have to leave my modesty at the door?

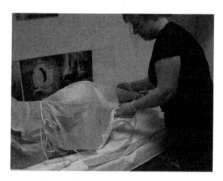

No, you really don't. All the colonic systems allow for a certain degree of privacy.

In Wellbeing Now, we use disposable underpants and disposable robes; we hope our clients feel that their privacy is protected. Many people have commented on how surprised they have been with the degree of privacy that was granted to them during the treatment.

Will I experience discomfort?

Well, as you know, a colonic session is not a facial. Sometimes, people feel queasy in the same way that they feel sick after an intensive workout in the gym, or if they've had a fast walk without having had a snack for a while and their blood sugar is low. There may be various reasons for feeling this way.

Sugar imbalance

The first reason is that you may indeed be getting low on sugar, if you have an excessive dependency on short fixes of glucose.

Leaky gut

The gut should be sealed from the rest of the body. Sometimes, the presence of allergens or certain medical conditions wear out the gut wall and increase its permeability - this is the condition known as 'leaky gut'.

If you suffer from a leaky gut, as the water soaks off the toxic wastes, some toxins escape and are picked up by your lymphatic and blood systems, causing a short-term liver overload, the effects of which are similar to those of food poisoning.

Brain oxygen supply

Another reason for having a 'sea-sick' feeling may be that as the water starts evacuating masses of wastes from the bowel, the body perceives the whole of the bowel as a site of emergency, and blood and endorphins rush to the area. As the blood supply within the large intestine increases, other parts of your body stop receiving their full share of oxygen.

The most oxygen-sensitive organ is, of course, the brain. The brain needs up to 40% of all oxygen used by the body. A good trick is to have something sweet during the treatment, which will immediately help boost the level of glucose in your body.

This seems to alleviate the discomfort, you become more relaxed, and it also makes it easier for you to focus on the treatment and to achieve a deeper cleanse.

Importance of breathing

The other way of dealing with the discomfort that you might be experiencing during the treatment is to focus on your breathing and on the positive effect that the treatment is having for you. Again, it is useful to compare colonic irrigation to a session with a personal trainer who pushes you quite hard, helping you to achieve your dream of a healthier, more sculptured body.

The bowel gets a workout

During the colonic treatment, your bowel gets what is virtually an endurance workout - the sets, the repetitions, working with weights (when water comes in) - so the bowel muscle does have to behave in the same way that muscles behave during a normal gym workout or a run.

When you set out for a run, at some point you really don't want to run; you really, really want to stop. At that point, the crux of the whole run, it is very important to focus on the goal. Why are you running? Maybe to be healthy, to have a greater lung capacity, to have a leaner body, to feel better or to get the adrenalin boost.

Visualizing in your mind the ultimate reason why you want to have a run keeps you going, and at some point you forget how bad it was at the start. Adrenalin kicks in, and you get great satisfaction out of your run.

A similar thing happens during a colonic treatment, but in a slightly different way. You need to focus on what is virtually a picture of health - a healthy looking, regularly contracting bowel. Imagine that the smooth intestinal walls have been cleared of all impurities, blood is flowing actively to the bowel and the bowel is absorbing nutrients from the good food that you have eaten.

This picture of health will help you deal with the discomfort during the treatment, and help achieve a more successful treatment.

How long will it last?

A colon hydrotherapy treatment can last between 35 minutes and about 65-70 minutes, which is the longest colonic procedure you should have. Otherwise, in the opinion of many colon hydrotherapists, the water in the body will put undue pressure on the kidneys.

The average duration of a colon hydrotherapy treatment is about 45 minutes. As mentioned above, your therapist might use some herbs, massage, heat, or change water temperature to promote bowel evacuation.

How do you know when the treatment is finished?

There are no hard and fast ways of telling that the treatment has finished. A lot depends on how comfortable you feel during the treatment, and on how well you and your bowel work together.

A caecum flush

If you are working well together, at some point in the treatment you should be able to observe a 'caecum flush', which looks a little bit like pea soup: this is the fresh stools that comes from the ascending colon, where it's just starting to form. It means that the water has gone all the way round and removed major wastes.

Following the caecum flush, you can expect the therapist to continue with the treatment for another couple of minutes;

the water will come out cleaner, with an occasional fluff of white, clean mucus.

Build-up of faecal matter

Sometimes there is a caecum flush at the beginning of a treatment. This may mean that the walls of the large intestine are covered in mucous faecal matter, and have become quite narrow.

The water is unable to soften this faecal matter at the start of the treatment, so it does not take long for it to pass through the narrow passage in the congested gut, all the way to the

WILL I LOSE WEIGHT ?....

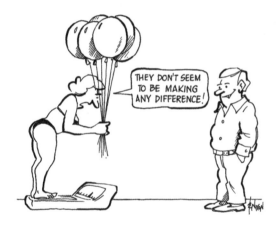

THEY DON'T SEEM TO BE MAKING ANY DIFFERENCE!

ileo-caecal valve. It is only later in the treatment that old matter starts soaking off the walls.

Sometimes, in cases of longstanding constipation, inflamed bowel or considerable nervousness, the first treatment can initially bring a disappointing outcome.

Nevertheless, some faecal matter will be moved during the first treatment, and you may achieve good results after it in terms of having somewhat larger and more regular bowel movements. So whatever result is achieved, it is going to bring some positive changes if you work with your body and help your bowel.

Will I lose weight?

You will lose wastes - some people lose more, some lose less. Some people absorb water and do not release it straight-away, especially if their bowel was dehydrated previously. The only proven way to lose weight is to move your body and eat good quality food in reasonable amounts.

Is the treatment dangerous?

As a client, you should know what risks are associated with any treatment that you decide to have, whether medical or non-medical. There are risks related to the use of aro-matherapy oils, nail varnishes, depilatory wax, and so on. Anything that can do good can also do harm if misused.

Colonics are used as a widespread detox treatment in the alternative medicine community. Like any other treatment, colonic irrigation involves risks. The main risks cited in the literature are related to contaminated equipment or water and damage to the bowel wall.

Your checklist

- Exposure to contaminated equipment is minimized when you go to a clinic that uses fully disposable kits. This is something you should ask for when booking your treatment. The more reliable and safety-conscious

clinics use medical disposal firms to collect
their disposable waste. No parts of disposable kits
should ever be re-used.

- To reduce the risk of water contamination, you should
  ask whether the clinic uses a system with a mechanical break required by some water authorities in the
  UK. Also ask how the mains water is filtered, because
  filtering water is another very important aspect of risk
  reduction.

- When using a closed system, the risk of bowel damage
  is extremely low when a professionally trained therapist
  inserts the speculum at the start of the treatment.
  Please note that insertion rules are different in the
  USA. The speculum is inserted to a maximum of 5-6
  centimetres (or just over 2 inches) and the therapist
  should always ask you how it feels. You may experience mild discomfort and/or mild irritation but NO
  SHARP PAIN. PAIN IS A SIGNAL TO STOP!

- In the open systems the client wriggles onto a small
  speculum, in a process known as self-insertion. Your
  colon hydrotherapist should guide you through the
  process to make sure it is safe.

- Whenever you book a treatment, make sure the clinic
  carries full public liability insurance. An insurance
  certificate should be available for your inspection or
  displayed on the premises.

How many treatments do I need?

Before you have had your first treatment, it isn't really
possible to say how many treatments you will require to
achieve substantial changes in your state of health and wellbeing.
Only after your first treatment will you know how it made you

feel and what effect it had on your digestive processes.

The treatments themselves are only a start, only a push in the right direction. What you do between treatments, how you change your diet, how you breathe and how you deal with stress, will play a major part in your self-improvement programme.

The basic rule

A very general basic rule is that healthy people under 30 years of age need a couple of treatments a year, unless they are competitive sportsmen or people who are under an inordinate amount of daily stress.

Generally, a couple of times a year for maintenance is great. As you get older, you may want to boost your system more often, and between the ages of 35 and 50 you might want to have the cleansing three or four times a year.

Those over the age of 50, as well as those who live and work in big cities, fly for business or pleasure, eat a lot of animal products, and, of course, smokers and drinkers might be recommended to have four to six treatments a year as maintenance. Again, it all depends on your health and how high you set your bar.

What should I do after the treatment?

As a general rule, relax, take it easy, don't engage into any strenuous activities, eat light, with the bulk of your nutrients coming from vegetables, fruit, juices and light proteins, and don't eat any spicy or rich foods at least for at least the next couple of days. Do not drink alcohol for 48 hours after the treatment.

What about probiotics?

Take probiotic supplements and eat live yoghurts. Eating fermented foods, such as live yoghurts, sauerkraut, miso and tofu, is extremely important after a colonic. The bowel is a naturally acidic environment. Probiotic bacteria survive best in lactic acid, and this is what fermented products help create.

Clients often ask me if it is worth buying the probiotic drinks that are sold in supermarkets. The reservation I have about these probiotic drinks is that they contain far too much sugar, and sugar should generally be avoided in the nutritional regime we recommend after treatment.

Eat fermented foods

Eating natural yoghurt and sauerkraut makes a lot more sense, because they are natural, living foods. If for some reason you can't eat live yoghurts or fermented foods, and you don't have access to probiotic supplements, a probiotic drink is certainly better than nothing.

The main thing you must remember is that you need to continue the cleansing process after the colonic treatment. Look after your body: it's the only place you've got to live.

Colonic irrigation and common digestive complaints

This book is about colonic irrigation as a tool in achieving digestive health; it is not specifically about digestive diseases, allergies and intolerances.

However, quite often I come across certain stereotypes of digestive ill-health in my daily practice and when advising clients.

The following is what my colleagues and I hear from many, many clients:

- My doctor told me I have got IBS. Can you treat IBS with colonics?

- I have *Candida* and I was told that if I have a colonic it might help.

- Can you see parasites in what comes out of me?

- Autointoxication: How long has this all been sitting in my bowel and poisoning me?

COLONIC IRRIGATION AND COMMON DIGESTIVE COMPLAINTS.....

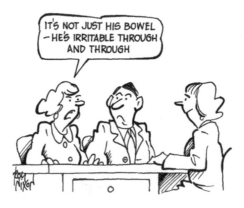

Irritable bowel syndrome (IBS)

IBS stands for the irritable bowel syndrome. It is not a disease; it is a condition caused by a combination of symptoms - i.e. a 'syndrome'.

It is quite hard to 'treat' IBS, because it is like 'treating' a headache: you need to find out where the headache comes from, and address the cause of the headache rather than the headache itself.

But there is no doubt that colonic irrigation is a great shortcut to IBS-free digestion. It can certainly alleviate the effects of IBS - bloatedness, discomfort, distended abdomen and alternating constipation and diarrhoea.

The real changes, however, will come after the colonic and between your treatments, in terms of more informed dietary choices, stress management and exercise. You will learn more in Part Four, 'Healthy Digestions and Weight Management', what choices you can make to relieve the symptoms of IBS.

Colonics and Candida

Candida is a much-abused word, like 'stress' or 'depression'. Some people, who suffer from digestive complaints, as well as some therapists and authors, blame *Candida* for every symptom of ill-health. 'Having *Candida* ' has become the equivalent to having the latest model of an Audi TT or a Gucci watch

- a

COLONIC IRRIGATION AND COMMON DIGESTIVE COMPLAINTS.....

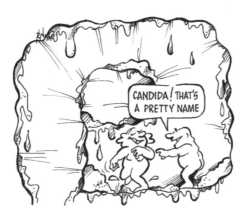

kind of a reverse fashion accessory.

Candida albicans is a yeast-like fungus that is normally present in the human body - in the normal flora of the mouth, skin, intestinal tract and vagina, alongside hundreds of thousands of other organisms. We have all got it.

If the body gets out of balance, for example because one's immunity is low, or there is too much sugar and alcohol in the digestive tract, *Candida* can become a health risk.

Generally, the excessive growth of yeasts, including *Candida*, is often an outcome of poor food and lifestyle choices, such as eating too many simple sugars, drinking too much alcohol and generally running yourself down, both physiologically and emotionally.

Colonic irrigation helps wash out a lot of the excessive fungus hanging around in the bowel. Sometimes the fungi come out like snowflakes, sometimes they are washed out with mucus, and sometimes they look like small scoops of cottage cheese in a bit of jelly. It is very therapeutic to see them going down the drain, and rewarding for both the client and therapist.

Colonic irrigation is a strong cleanse, akin to spring-cleaning a house or clearing out a garden. As we all know, if you do not maintain order in your house or garden, things will quickly return to the way they were.

The main thing to remember is that *Candida* does not 'attack' or 'invade' - it comes from within, so to get rid of *Candida* you need to review your dietary and lifestyle choices. Again, read Part Four.

Colonics and parasites

Unlike yeasts, parasites are true invaders. They attack everyone; but for the most part, people with strong immune systems can resist these attacks.

During colonic irrigation treatments, it is quite difficult to see parasites in faeces, because they are small and normally impossible to see in the flood of wastes without magnification.

The only parasites that can be seen and easily identified are bits of tapeworms, and even then it is quite rare to see a whole dead tapeworm.

Colonic irrigation may help clean the bowel of parasites, and may weaken their larvae by strengthening the immune system.

We need to bear in mind though, that colonics may not be able to alleviate parasitic infections outside the bowel, in muscles or connective tissue.

Generally, if you suspect you have got a parasitic infection, the best thing to do is to see a holistic medical practitioner, who will advise on further tests and possible treatments.

The concept of autointoxication

Autointoxication is, in my opinion, another hugely over-used buzzword. In colon cleansing circles it is described as a self-poisoning process through the re-absorption of your own bowel toxins, a.k.a 'slow death'.

Often clients who see a lot of wastes coming out ask: 'How long has this all been sitting in me? Can it be years? Am I a toxic dump?'

I don't think so: if the situation was that bad, most of us would be dead already!

There is no doubt that carrying around a lot of waste is not a good idea. Birds don't do it, bees don't do it, cats, dogs, cows and horses don't do it - they drop it down, bring it out, do whatever it takes to get rid of it.

Wastes wear out the body

So what about humans? Well, I have seen people who have bowel movements twice a month while taking in around 1,500 calories a day. They don't look particularly healthy, but they drive themselves to treatments and back and survive the trip. So there must be a mechanism in the human body that enables it to perform an amazing over-the-top balancing act in order to survive.

You have read a couple of pages earlier the story of one of my clients who had not had any bowel movements for almost two months, and she still managed to come for a treatment with her husband. She is a living testament to the amazing power of adaptation that we all possess.

Having said that, I first thought she was about 20 years older than her husband. It was only a couple of weeks later, after her bowel movements had returned and she came back for her second and final treatment with her husband again, that I realized they were around the same age. The change in her appearance was remarkable.

Make sure you are in the right gear

I believe that if we don't evacuate through the channels that are designed for evacuation, the body will find another way. I repeatedly see constipated clients with bad breath, unhealthy skin, acid reflux and low energy levels. They 'poo' through their bad skin, bad breath, incomplete digestion and poor blood quality.

I am convinced that when the bowel shuts down, the body is forced to break the wastes into minute components that weasel their way into the blood, skin and breath - a process that on a regular basis, systematically wears out the body.

Would you drive on a motorway on a Sunday night in second gear? You would not, because it would 'kill' your car. Well, to put it in simple terms, if you don't eliminate wastes regularly, you always drive in second gear.

Colon hydrotherapy and related treatments

Colon hydrotherapy is a great stand-alone treatment, but it works even more effectively when combined with other educational, bodywork, health and emotional awareness tools. For the last couple of years, we have been offering clients treatments that we call 'colonic combos'.

A colonic combo is a combination of colonic irrigation and another treatment. The following briefly describes the treatments we in Wellbeing Now include in colonic combos and the rationale behind our decisions to offer our clients these combinations.

Colonics and visual medicine self-awareness tools

Enabling treatments

The first group of treatments combines colonics with education and health awareness tools - live blood microscopy, kinesiology, iridology and naturopathy, including tongue, nail and skin analysis.

I call this category of treatments 'enabling treatments', because they give clients a tool they can use to enhance their own state of health.

Live blood microscopy

Live blood microscopy allows you to watch your live blood on screen. One of my teachers, Dr Sanjay Chaudhuri, describes live blood microscopy as visual medicine, and I think this is an extremely appropriate name for it. You can watch your red and white blood cells and plasma on the computer or TV screen and assess their condition.

Clients who come to live blood microscopy sessions can see very clearly if their blood cells are suffering from environmental damage, oxidative damage, lack of hydration or congestion. Observing your own living blood becomes a great visual aid in the quest for better health, and, in combination with colon hydrotherapy, which is also very visual, achieves very good results in a short space of time.

Kinesiology

Kinesiology works on the body's energy circuits and involves testing large muscles, as well as the body's responses to food, chemical, herbal and homeopathic remedies. The main premise of kinesiology is that the body has innate wisdom, and it knows what it needs.

I do believe in the inner wisdom of the body and in its intuition. Kinesiolgy is a great self-assessment tool for people with a strongly developed 'gut feeling' and self-awareness.

Iridology

Iridology is art-based naturopathic science. Iridologists can look into your eyes with a magnifying glass and read imbalances of your internal organs from what they see in your eyes. Many colon hydrotherapists use iridology as an initial diagnostic tool in their practice, and it works very well for a lot of practitioners.

Being a good iridologist involves a certain degree of spirituality, as well as a sound knowledge of the body's anatomy and physiology.

If you have an opportunity to have a colonic treatment and a consultation with an experienced colon hydrotherapist and iridologist, it is certainly worth going for it. The knowledge and education you receive in the course of your consultation will be invaluable to you.

Naturopathy

My favourite combination is of colonic irrigation with a naturopathic consultation. An ideal naturopathic consultation would involve live blood microscopy, elements of kinesiology, some iridology, a nutritional review and a tongue, nails and skin analysis.

In Wellbeing Now we do a half-day treatment and diagnostic crash course, which includes all these tools and a full colonic treatment. It is amazing how well this package works! We've seen people change their whole attitude towards their body in a heartbeat, when they have opened all their channels, both physical and emotional, to self-improvement.

Colonics and bodywork treatments

The next group of treatments that I value greatly is bodywork treatments. Colonics is a truly holistic procedure; it involves your brain, your body and your emotions. It is complemented extremely well by massage, reflexology and body wraps.

The power of human touch

All these forms of bodywork have a great power of touch. Many of us, children of the twenty-first century, suffer from what I call 'an acute touch deficiency', or 'Vitamin T deficiency' - a kind of twenty-first century emotional scurvy.

While massage, aromatherapy, reflexology and wraps have undoubtedly many energy-enhancing and detoxification benefits, they mainly address our touch deficit disorder and our over-the-top stress levels. They make us feel loved, cared for and nurtured.

Together with the great cleansing and liberating effect of colonic treatment, they make a very good start to engaging in a more wholesome lifestyle, in which you value yourself more as a person.

Colon hydrotherapy and emotional balancing therapies

Sometimes colon hydrotherapy addresses such long-term complaints as irritable bowel syndrome or constipation, which are caused by outstanding emotional issues waiting for closure.

To help our clients resolve these issues, we offer colon hydrotherapy treatments combined with hypnotherapy and journey therapy.

Journey therapy and hypnotherapy

Journey therapy uncovers unresolved emotions from the past that get trapped in the physical tissues of our bodies and restrict our current lives. Hypnotherapy is another device for positive change that uses our imagination as a tool. Both enable us to free ourselves from fears and restrictions that sometimes govern our most important decisions.

Colonics is also an extremely liberating treatment at a deeply physical level.

The combination of colonics and emotional release treatments is sometimes extremely effective in resolving long-standing emotional conflicts and issues and reaching the closure that is so badly needed.

Advice to colon hydrotherapists

If you are a colon hydrotherapist reading these lines, thinking, 'but I'm not a trained journey therapist and I'm not a trained hypnotherapist and I can't take money and time out of my practice to go and retrain', then start by honing your listening skills.

Start by letting people talk, don't pre-judge, don't invade their space, just let them express themselves, because if they do, they let go and you have one satisfied customer after another.

As a therapist, you will probably realize at some point that you need to learn additional skills that will be important in your practice and when you do, you will go and acquire them.

 The colonic process was physically and emotionally difficult for me; However, the combination of hypnotherapy and colonic irrigation was both powerful and incredibly healing. I was able to relax and allow both processes to flow their way.

Colonics and exercise

Another of my favourite combinations is colonics plus exercise. My two favourite types of exercise are yoga and stretching.

Ernest Coates, who used to be Chairman of Friends of Yoga International, is responsible for stretching me well past my physical boundaries. He helped me realize at a very practical, four-hooves-on-the-ground level, that it is not the body that runs the brain, and it is not the brain that runs the body, but it is the balanced spirit that runs both.

I have based my bowel therapy exercises that you will find at the end of the book on Earnest Coates' yogic toxic cleansing routine described by him in great detail in his book 'Living Yoga', the details of which are in the book list.

The 'bottom line'

The 'bottom line' is that colonic irrigation is just one of the tools.

We all should all have a number of tools in our health toolkit. The most important tool for some people is nutrition, for some it is exercise, for others it is treatments.

All you need to find is a balance between the demands of the twenty-first century, such as having to combine numerous roles, being what we are, and finding out why we are here and what the whole purpose of our existence is.

The book that you are reading does not specifically address these questions, but it doesn't mean that you should not. In fact, if you are reading this book because you have some really bad digestive problems, some of the questions you should probably ask are: What am I doing? What am I doing right? What am I doing wrong? Am I focused? Am I balanced? Am I living true to my calling? Is every day of my life a rewarding day?

If you want to have more energy, be more satisfied with your life, manage your cravings, or if you want to have more control over your eating and drinking, feel less bloated or less constipated, may be these are the questions that you need to address.

Colonic irrigation is a tool that helps you address these questions is a very physical, direct way. Here is how it can happen in practice.

Anna's journey

Here is an interesting case study that demonstrates how everything comes together. This is the story of a woman who came to us for an eight-day detox in October 2005. I'll call her Anna.

Before Anna came to us we had had quite a few telephone conversations with her. We understood that she needed to change something in her life. She was middle-aged, with some personal problems, taking an array of medications, but with a fantastic spirit that took a lot of battering but was still hanging in there.

The treatment plan

Anna's detoxification and rejuvenation package involved four colonic irrigation treatments, hypnotherapy and emotional balancing, massages, wraps, a couple of powerful rejuvenating facials, lymphatic drainage, live blood microscopy, naturopathy and physical exercise.

She did a lot of walking, mild rebounding and stretching. She was juicing daily, did not eat any processed foods, but instead ate only very simple foods, such as grains, sprouts, fruit and vegetables, live yoghurt, cottage cheese and clean proteins (organic eggs, fish and chicken).

Generally, she took time out to rebalance herself, and find who she was and where this absolutely overwhelming desire to change her life originated.

A difficult start

When Shoela Detsios, our naturopathic therapist, first took Anna's live blood sample, the day after Anna started with us, she did not quite know what to say.

Anna's red blood cells were stuck together and heavily stacked; there was a lot of gunk in her plasma and the blood was showing massive environmental damage and lack of balance. Shoela even took a couple of samples, to make sure that what she had seen was true, and every sample brought the same disheartening result.

We decided to take it slowly, one step at a time. Kim Verhoeven who specializes in colonics and emotional therapies worked on re-establishing the connection between the body and the emotional self of our client.

Anna's colonics

It is interesting to follow the story of the colonics that Anna had with us. The first colonic was good for someone who had never had one before. Anna had a good release and she started to relax.

Anna's second colonic was scheduled immediately after her power walk with me. During the power walk we addressed some emotional issues, including her basic fears and insecurities.

One of Anna's major insecurities revolved around being honest with her parents about her emotional, physical and financial conditions. She found the idea of 'coming out' to her parents and revealing to them that she was broke, emotionally exhausted and not able to enjoy life absolutely terrifying.

When Anna returned to the practice for her colonic, she was unable to release, because her whole being, every single cell in her body, was terrified of even thinking about confronting her parents. Instead, Kim conducted her initial session of hypnotherapeutic preparation for an emotional and physical release.

The third colonic was a hypno-colonic and it produced absolutely outstanding results.

This is what Anna said immediately afterwards:

'The colonic process was physically and emotionally difficult for me; however, the combination of hypnotherapy and colonic irrigation was both powerful and incredibly healing. I was able to relax and allow both processes to flow their way.'

This was a fantastic result for us, and we carried on.

A great outcome

When Shoela took Anna's blood sample on the last day of her detox break, we actually couldn't believe the extent of the difference. Textbooks say that it takes 120 days to change the blood. So when we started with Anna we were quite realistic about how much we would achieve in a week.

On the whole, the outcome of our work with Anna was so amazing that Shoela couldn't believe her eyes when she looked at the blood samples. She took another couple of samples to make sure they were true samples - and yes, it was the real stuff.

Here you can see the comparison, judge it for yourself.

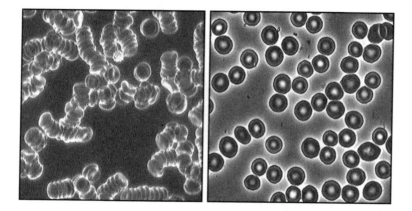

The change

This is what Anna wrote:

I arrived here seven days ago desperate and exhausted, praying for a miracle to heal my sick and weary body, and I will be leaving not only physically but emotionally cleansed. My journey has been painful, but with the love support and compassion of all at Wellbeing Now, both gentle and manageable but most of all safe. I will leave feeling clean, pure and rejuvenated having dealt with the issues of the past that were dragging me down and destroying my very being, knowing that I have been given skills and knowledge to manage my own life with confidence and grace when I leave. I am on the beginning of a new journey and the joy of getting to know myself again.

I will certainly return to the nourishing womblike environment that is Wellbeing Now. Even though we are cosseted and protected here, we are given the skills to grow up and grow strong. Consequently we are able to follow our path through life, with confidence, anticipation and pleasure.

You have taken me to the core of my being, and showed me the beauty within. You have saved my life and given me hope and purpose for the future and for that I thank you.

The colonic process was physically and emotionally difficult for me; However, the combination of hypnotherapy and colonic irrigation was both powerful and incredibly healing. I was able to relax and allow both processes to flow their way.

Thank you for your strength, your tenacity, your loving focus and honesty.

Thank you for your sensitivity, understanding, sharing your bravery, courage and fragility with me.

Thank you for sharing your wisdom, your love of life and the joy of bouncing.

Thank you for your beauty, your inner peace, your grace and perfect love that has flown from your fingertips into my body.

Thank you for helping me to trust again. I leave you knowing that I have found my own space.

Summary: your road map to colonic irrigation

- Colon hydrotherapy is not a new procedure. The first recorded mention of colon cleansing is as early as 1500 B.C.

- The benefits of colon hydrotherapy all originate from removing stored wastes from the large intestine. The goals you can achieve are to:

  - remove the waste, the irritants and allergy triggers

  - rehydrate the bowel

  - repair the gut wall

  - replace digestants and rebalance the bowel flora

  - rebuild the gut-brain connection

  - restore the bowel function

  - re-educate the owner of the bowel

- No two people are the same, and it is important for you to understand why you personally have opted to have colon hydrotherapy treatments.

- If you are a healthy person, with a good diet and regular bowel movements, you can expect to have a short and comfortable treatment.

- Treatments can last between 35 and 65-70 minutes, which is the longest procedure you should have. The average duration of a colonic treatment is about 45 minutes.

- Make sure you use a clinic that is fully insured, uses disposable equipment, has colonic devices that are Water Board-compliant, and uses a water-filtering procedure. Clinics using special firms to dispose of their waste are likely to be more reliable and safety-conscious. No disposable parts should ever be re-used.

- The risk of bowel damage is extremely low when the therapist inserts the speculum at the start of the treatment. You may experience mild discomfort or mild irritation, but NO SHARP PAIN. PAIN IS A SIGNAL TO STOP! Please note that insertion rules in the UK and the USA are different.

- If you suffer from severe constipation and some other digestive conditions, you may need to have a few colonic treatments with only short intervals between them.

- We all need to have a number of tools in our health toolkit. Colonic irrigation is an extremely effective tool, especially when combined with other naturopathic treatments and lifestyle changes.

PART THREE

THE BIGGER PICTURE:
NUMBER TWO EXPLAINED

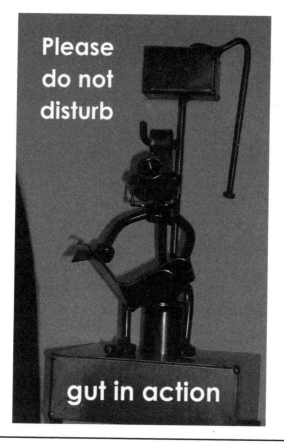

PART THREE: THE BIGGER PICTURE
NUMBER TWO EXPLAINED

Seven important bowel functions

Winning the poo

Seven habits of a highly effective bowel

What could slight imperfections in my bowel movements mean?

Improving the quality of your eliminations

Summary: your road map to winning the poo

Seven important bowel functions

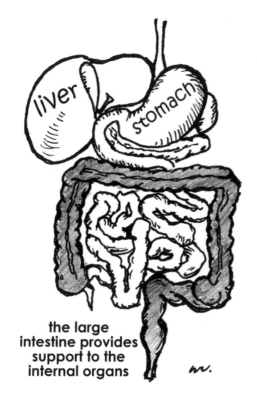

the large intestine provides support to the internal organs

Everyone needs a healthy bowel. Open any atlas of human anatomy and you will probably realize that the bowel, or the large intestine, that is about as long as you are tall, frames all the internal organs of your abdominal cavity. It supports them and keeps them in place.

If a section of the large intestine is misplaced, for example if the transverse colon prolapsed, it would exert excessive pressure on the small intestine, the reproductive organs and the bladder, while the organs that are resting on the transverse colon (the liver, stomach and kidneys) would lose valuable support.

The large bowel specializes in environmentally friendly disposal and recycling of digestive wastes.

> **SEVEN IMPORTANT BOWEL FUNCTIONS**
>
> 1. Supporting and massaging the organs of the abdominal cavity.
> 2. Recycling water and nutrients back into circulation.
> 3. Producing serotonin, our mood-regulating neurotransmitter.
> 4. Producing vitamin K and some vitamins of the B group.
> 5. Producing stool-fermenting enzymes and fermenting wastes.
> 6. Supporting the body's immune system and organizing protection against pathogens.
> 7. Eliminating digestive wastes.

Waste removal

The whole waste removal process is based on the activities of the intestinal flora, which manufacture faeces, and smooth muscle contractions, which propel the faeces towards the anus.

Muscle contractions take place in sections. As a short section of the bowel contracts, it propels its contents into the next section. The next section will then contract and either move the contents back into the previous section of the bowel or move it forward. This contractile movement, called peristalsis, is necessary for the bowel to accomplish many of its essential functions.

The bowel needs to absorb about 1.5 litres of liquid a day from the chyme - the digested food mix that it receives from the small intestine.

As the chyme moves along, gut bacteria release important enzymes that help ferment the wastes.

After the remaining nutrients and excess water have been re-absorbed and the wastes have been fully fermented, the smooth muscle propels the wastes towards the rectum and anus, through which they are going to be eliminated in a movement called mass peristalsis.

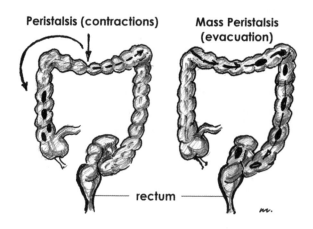

Peristalsis (contractions) Mass Peristalsis (evacuation)

rectum

Winning the poo

Respect your intestinal flora

Our large intestine or bowel accommodates between 200 and 500 different colonies of bacteria. Each one of us is a host to a whole sealed eco-system, and no two eco-systems are the same.

Here are some pretty amazing facts that can be found on the website of the Society for General Microbiology, www.microbiologyonline.org.uk:

'There are more microbial cells in our bodies than there are human cells.

In fact 95% of all the cells in the body are bacteria, mainly living in the digestive tract. There are more bacteria in the colon than the total number of people who have ever lived.

Everyone has about 1 kg in weight of bacteria in their gut. Each gram of faeces contains 100,000,000,000 microbes. Human adults excrete their own weight in faecal bacteria every year.'

Our cooperation with the beneficial bacteria in our gut appears to be a result of billions of years of evolution.

There is a lot of research on gut bacteria, showing that the lawful inhabitants of the large intestine not only help eliminate wastes, but also act as the most effective immune barrier for the whole body, destroy invading pathogens, manufacture vitamins, and provide the body with other services that are only now coming to light.

Endangered species

Great dangers to this eco-system come from the outside - in the form of undesirable pathogens, including harmful bacteria and parasites, which would compete with the beneficial bacteria for space and food.

However, even greater dangers come from our food and lifestyle choices: excessive sugar, alcohol, cigarettes, antibiotics, painkillers, other prescription drugs, illegal drugs, and processed foods are among the greatest enemies of the beneficial bacteria.

If you want to keep your gut healthy, make sure you eat

fresh vegetables, sprouted pulses, grains and s
fermented products, such as kefir and sauerkraut,
gut can maintain the acidic environment that helps destroy
pathogens. You can find more information on healthy eating
systems in Part Four.

The great debate

So, one of the bowel's main functions is to eliminate digestive wastes.

At some point in time, many of us have wondered: how
much we should eliminate and how often?

The mainstream medicine camp says that you go when
you go; if you don't go, don't worry too much about it. The
alternative view is that you need to go after every meal.

One extreme

On the one hand, Encyclopaedia Britannica states in one
of its articles that there is nothing wrong with constipation and
that faeces have been proven to stay in the bowel for over a
year without any harmful effects on the bowel's owner:

*'Faeces are normally removed from the body one or two times
daily. They may become impacted as a result of growths in the rectum,
obstructions in the colon, deficiencies in diet, or constipation.
Autointoxication, or poisoning by toxins produced by stored faecal
material, is a myth. Several cases have been reported in which faecal
material has been retained in the intestine for a year or more without
suffering any bad effects other than extra burden of carrying 25 to 45
kilograms (60 to 100 pounds) of faecal material'* (15th Edition,
Volume 4, Page 710).

The other extreme

On the other hand we know the opinion of famous 20th century naturopaths Dr Jensen and Dr Kellogg, who spent decades of their professional careers saying that if you don't eliminate your wastes daily and preferably 2 or 3 times a day, you are in danger of suffering from major degenerative diseases.

They have said that health is virtually stored in the colon, and, consequently, disease also begins in the colon. Dr Bernard Jensen, in his 'Guide to better bowel care' stated that:

'Constipation is often referred to by those who have studied it as 'the modern plague'. Indeed, I consider it the greatest present-day internal danger to health. Intestinal toxaemia and autointoxication are direct result of intestinal constipation. Constipation contributes to the lowering of the body's resistance, predisposing the body to many acute illnesses and the initiation of many degenerative and chronic processes. Constipation indirectly cripples and kills more people in our country than almost any other single disease condition having to do with deficient function'. (Avery, 1999, p.46)

A quirky note on wastes and fat

The bowel can store wastes, while the rest of the body can store quite a lot of fat. Some of the fat is stored for energy. However, there are people who have far too much stored energy - in other words who are grossly overweight.

These people pay higher insurance premiums, because the mainstream medical community understands very well that people with that amount of stored energy are a walking and talking actuarial risk.

It is quite bizarre, though, that the same sort of logic does not apply to those people who carry around kilos of stored wastes.

People who empty their bowels only twice a month never get disqualified from anything, and never get to pay more, because society doesn't consider it as something it will end up paying for. Nevertheless, colon disorders, and especially colon cancer, cost society probably as much as obesity.

I would not be surprised if in 10 years' time questions concerning the body's eliminative functions become routine in all medical insurance assessments.

How much poo is good enough?

At the end of the day, we all need to understand 'how much is good enough?'

Let us do some simple maths. An 'average' adult eats about 2 kg of food a day. In a healthy eater, the liquid content of this food should be about 70%, or around 1.4 kg. So, on a healthy day, we eat about 500-600g of what could be described as solid foods. The body will manage to get some liquid out of these solid foods too. It will obtain its nutrients by almost fully breaking up fats and proteins; it will convert carbohydrates into glucose to use as energy, and then it will try to remove the remainder as wastes.

It would be reasonable to assume that around a quarter, by weight, of all the solid food that we eat will need to be eliminated.

What's in the poo?

This will be some soluble and all of the insoluble fibre which serves as a cleansing agent for the body, as well as the indigestible parts of proteins and fats that the body has decided not to use or that it is unable to use for any reason. This will also include the agents that you might be intolerant of, or allergic to, and so on.

So this alone gives us around 100 to 150 g of semi-solid wastes.

In addition, as the fibres and wastes pass through the stomach and through the small intestine into the large intestine, they will also collect and mop up all the dead cells.

It is worth remembering that the cells of the stomach work really, really hard in a very acid environment. They are renewed every 4 days. The working conditions of the cells in the small intestine are not much better, and they have a very short life span too: they serve their purpose and die.

There will also be plenty of decommissioned red blood cells which are converted into bilirubin (the main component of bile that breaks up fats) and then eventually into stercobilinogen, which gives the faeces their characteristic rusty-brown colour.

Also, the stool comprises dead bowel flora, parasites and other gut buddies that make their home in the large intestine.

Find your own benchmark

So it would not be unreasonable to eliminate somewhere in the region of 200 g of faeces a day, if our food intake is about 2 kg, less if we eat less and more if we eat more.

The factor that will have the biggest effect on the volume of eliminations is the amount of fibre and water in our diet. Someone who eats grains and vegetables and drinks a sufficient amount of water will eliminate more than someone who is on a high-protein and low-carbohydrate diet.

It is also worth remembering that elimination of stored wastes, both food and non-food in origin, will continue even if the food intake is minimal, for example during periods of cleansing or detoxification.

Don't put up with poor eliminations!

As you already know, people who don't eat enough fibre or whose diet is too dry, as well as those who 'bottle up' emotions and stress, won't eliminate as much.

However, just because these people don't eliminate a certain amount of stools, it doesn't mean that they don't produce as much composted waste. All it means is that the body's waste removal plant does not get enough fibre-based fuel, and therefore it does not have enough power to be able to get rid of it.

You will still need to get rid of the dead blood cells, the dead cells from your stomach and your gut, the bits you are allergic to and other undesirable elements. The large bowel is storage medium and it can put up with a lot. The question is: do you want to put up with it?

So how can I tell whether my bowel is working properly?

The first sign is the call of nature. Do you know when it is time to open your bowels? How does your brain know that your body needs to eliminate wastes?

Do you have a reasonably established pattern? For example, do go to the toilet on arising, or do you regularly go to the toilet after breakfast? Do you miss an occasional day, but the next day you will have a bowel evacuation that is slightly larger and slightly more satisfying than usual? Then, your bowel seems to be doing its job.

If, when you have finished your bowel evacuation, you have a feeling that nothing is left in the lower gut, and after getting off the toilet you feel relieved and lighter, it means that your body is doing its job.

On the other hand, your digestive system is not working at full efficiency if
- you feel heavy and bloated;
- you feel hardness in your bowels;
- you go daily, but never get the satisfaction of the job well done;
- you constantly have this niggling sensation of unfinished business.

Seven habits of a highly effective bowel

SEVEN HABITS OF A HIGHLY EFFECTIVE BOWEL

1. You are aware of the call of nature.
2. The feeling that you need to open your bowels is strong, but not overwhelming.
3. When you sit on the toilet, the release is easy; you do not need to 'help it out'.
4. The smell is faint rather than overpowering.
5. Straining is minimal.
6. There is no feeling of 'unfinished business'.
7. There is a feeling of comfortable physical and emotional relief.

What should 'it' look like?

If 'it' is nice and healthy, it should look like a soft sausage, the colour should be light to medium brown, slightly golden and shiny. The texture should be that of peanut butter. Being slightly acidic, 'it' should float first and sink soon afterwards without leaving 'skid marks' when you flush 'it'.

Obviously there are variations. If you eat a lot of grains, 'it' will be slightly looser and the sausage will break in the middle, leaving a rough edge. If you eat lots of leafy green vegetables, 'it' will look quite dark.

Beetroot will make your stools a kind of crimson red, while charcoal will make it dark. Iron supplements can make your stools harder and darker.

By the way, iron supplements can make some people constipated. If you are wondering why you are constipated on a good diet, sufficient liquid intake and good level of exercise, and if you are taking a multivitamin with iron or an iron supplement, try, as an experiment, to change your multivitamin to one without iron. Note whether this condition changes.

THE BEST TYPE OF 'IT'

Generally, if you eat a reasonably varied diet, with enough fibre, 'it' should come out as a golden brown sausage, up to 200 g in weight, a floater that leaves no skid marks. 'It' should be almost smell free.

Looking at your creation

When we are babies and haven't yet learned to talk, our mothers can tell if we are happy, unhappy, content or miserable just by looking at our poo. As we grow up, our poo becomes something intensely private, a 'closed-door' subject for most people, especially women.

However, if you want to know how your digestive system is working, all you need to do is look at your poo. A picture, as the saying goes, speaks a thousand words.

The transit time

The size and shape of your stools indicate how long the food has spent in your digestive tract. This is called the 'transit time'. The transit time in a healthy large bowel should be between 18 and 36 hours from the moment the food is eaten, to the moment the waste is eliminated.

In the UK, the average transit time is at least twice as long - 54 to 72 hours. Longer transit times may be associated with low energy levels, bad skin, congested blood, decreased immunity and degenerative diseases, including colon cancer.

To check your transit time, eat some fresh or boiled beetroot and note the date and time, and then see how long it takes for your stools to become crimson-red in colour.

Alternatively, you can take some charcoal tablets and check how long it takes for the stools to darken up.

The Bristol Stool Form Scale

To help you identify how your digestive system works, and whether it gets rid of the wastes in an efficient manner, the official Bristol Stool Form Scale divides stools into seven distinct types in terms of size, shape and colour.

- Dry with hard lumps or clumps: CONSTIPATION.

- Like lumpy sausage: CONSTIPATION.

- Like sausage with surface cracks: HEALTHY, VERY SLIGHTLY DEHYDRATED.

- Long smooth surface. Normal, good colour, quick exit, and easy to clean: HEALTHY.

- In blobs with well-defined margins: HEALTHY.

- Fluffy with ragged edges: BORDERING ON DIARRHOEA.

- Watery with no solids: DIARRHOEA.

The size and shape of the stools indicate the transit time through the digestive tract. The colour can tell you how good your digestion is and alert you to other changes concerning your wellness.

The Bristol Stool Form Scale

Type 1	Separate hard lumps, like nuts
Type 2	Sausage-like, but lumpy
Type 3	Like a sausage but with cracks in the surface
Type 4	Like a sausage or snake, smooth and soft
Type 5	Soft blobs with clear cut edges
Type 6	Fluffy pieces with ragged edges, a mushy stool
Type 7	Watery, no solid pieces

What could slight imperfections in my bowel movements mean?

You may not be aware for quite a while of anything going wrong in your bowel: it is not designed to send progress reports to the central nervous system until the condition is established and your bowel is unable to cope with it alone.

Therefore, any discomfort relayed by the bowel to the brain is a serious cry for help and should not be ignored.

Skid marks

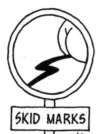

Skid marks are often present after a night on the town, and they appear when passing soft stools that leave a slightly burning sensation after being released.

Alcoholic drinks contain salts, and are often accompanied by meals high in salt, proteins and fat. This draws excessive amounts of water from outside the bowel wall into the bowel itself, making the stools heavier and reducing the transit time.

Shorter transit time may cause malabsorption, often wasting valuable nutrients.

Skid marks combined with sticky, foul-smelling and greasy stools can be a sign of fat malabsorption in the small intestine, due to poor bile action, or stomach acid deficiency that affects the digestion of proteins in the stomach.

Greasy stools

If stools are fatty and hard to flush, it means that fats are not being properly broken down - due either to bile insufficiency or

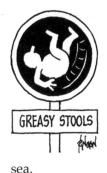

GREASY STOOLS

to excessive consumption of fats, especially of animal origin.

If, trying to lose weight, you have taken some fat-blocking tablets, you will have seen that the toilet water, once you've had a bowel movement, is full of orange-slick puddles which are reminiscent of an oil slick in the sea.

This is unfortunately what these fat blockers do - they pass the fat straight into your bowel. You may have soft evacuations, because the fat is a great lubricant, but these pills can wreak havoc with your bowel flora.

It takes quite some time for the bowel ecosystem to recover from the effects of fat blockers.

Anal itching

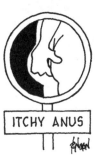

ITCHY ANUS

Most adults experience anal itching, the soreness around the anus and the irresistible desire to scratch at some point in their life.

The itching itself is a sign of something going wrong somewhere in the body.

Sometimes the cause is simple and local: wearing clothes that are too tight; dry skin or, on the contrary, too much moisture on the skin; even sweating or using shower gels that can cause a skin allergy.

Occasionally the causes are found in overusing laxative preparations, taking some antibiotics (especially if they cause diarrhoea); or being prone to psoriasis or eczema.

Itching could also be caused by dysbiosis, which results in excessive yeast production in the bowel (the best known manifestation of this condition is *Candida albicans*), or by infections, especially by worms or other parasites.

Finally, the dietary 'culprits' that cause dysbiosis and itching often are coffee and other drinks containing caffeine, nuts, popcorn, tomatoes, chocolates and sometimes fruit.

Light-coloured greyish stools

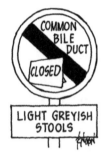

Light-coloured and greyish stools can be indicative of anaemia (shortage of iron in red blood cells), gallstones or other blockages in the bile duct, as well as of insufficient production of bile by the body.

White chalk-like stools

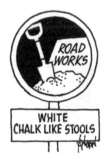

White chalk-like stools normally result from a combination of factors: low-fibre diet high in fat and processed foods, anaemia and severe dysbiosis that is often caused by excessive or long-term use of prescription drugs, appetite suppressants, street narcotics and laxatives. All this virtually brings the colon to a standstill.

Apparently, the autopsy on Elvis Presley showed that his colon was approximately twice the normal diameter - around 12-13 cm (or 5 inches) compared to the 'norm' of 5.5 to 6.5 cm (about 2.5 inches) and full of compacted chalk-like faeces.

Elvis was notorious as an unhealthy eater, who was prescribed *'the constellation of uppers, downers, laxatives, nar-*

cotics, hormones and shots that kept Elvis going through the last decade of his life.' (Doctor Feelgood. The Observer Magazine, 11 August 2002).

At the time of his death he was suffering from an enlarged colon.

Gassy (smelly) stools

Often gassy, smelly stools are the evidence of lactose intolerance (lactose is found primarily in milk). This means that the body is deficient in lactase, an enzyme that speeds up the breakdown of lactose.

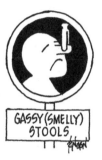

GASSY (SMELLY) STOOLS

These stools can also be caused by a bacterial infection or dysbiosis.

Sometimes gassy smelly stools are caused by overdoing one type of food, especially high-fibre vegetables, such as onions or artichokes, or beans and pulses.

On the other hand, gas can also be caused by the excessive consumption of fatty animal foods combined with stomach acid or bile deficiency.

Mucus in stools

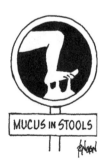

MUCUS IN STOOLS

If you have mucus in your stools, this can also mean several things. There might be an agent that your body is intolerant to, and the bowel lining has secreted excess mucus to try to eliminate it.

On the other hand, it might mean that you are eating a disproportionate amount of proteins and fats, especially of animal origin, also including milk, yoghurts, fromage frais and cheeses.

Some people process milk products, animal proteins and fats better than others. If you regularly consume high amounts of proteins and you don't find any mucus in your stools, then your body seems to be coping.

It is worth remembering though, that most people are historically and biologically conditioned to eat fewer proteins and more grains, vegetables and pulses.

If you consistently find mucus in your stool, try to eliminate animal proteins for a while and increase your fibre intake, and see if the situation improves.

The bowel will produce excessive mucus mostly for its own protection, or in order to increase the lubrication of the bowel wall, and to wrap up and help eliminate undesirable wastes. It could be caused by dysbiosis, bacterial infections, and obstructions in the bowel, parasites, haemorrhoids and a multitude of other things.

Blood-containing mucus in your stools is a good reason to have your stools checked professionally.

Goat pellets

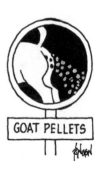

Goat pellets (also known as 'rabbit droppings') are normally a sign of constipation caused by dehydration.

If you don't eat enough fibre, which serves as a bulking agent, and don't drink enough liquid, which helps increase the

GOAT PELLETS

weight of the waste, your stools may be small in size and very compacted.

Sometimes people have a good diet, but still produce goat pellets. This could be a sign of adrenal exhaustion, of an emotional blockage or of high levels of suppressed stress and anxiety that increase acidity in the body.

Bits of undigested food

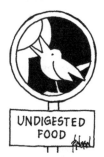

UNDIGESTED
FOOD

If you have discernible bits of food in your stools, it might mean that you are not chewing your food properly.

It may also mean the bacterial colonies that live in your small and large bowels are not doing a very good job. Or it may be that you are not producing enough of the enzymes that speed up food assimilation by the body.

Some foods are notoriously harder to digest than others. A lot of people do not digest tomato, potato and apple skins, seeds or nuts, sweet corn and popcorn.

Peeling your fruit and vegetables and not eating the skins, making sure that sweetcorn or popcorn are chewed properly and grinding your seeds and nuts shortly before eating should help your digestive system and assist in nutrient absorption and assimilation.

Straining and constipation

Straining is a sign of constipation.

If you have a bowel movement less often than every day with an occasional day off, then you are almost certainly suf-

STRAINING & CONSTIPATION

fering from habitual constipation. It means, in simple terms, that dead stuff is not getting out through the bowel.

Straining means that the stool is too dry or dehydrated to come out on its own. It irritates the nerve endings in the lower bowel enough to create an urge, but there is insufficient moisture and bulk in the stool to build momentum for an easy evacuation. It may also be indicative of a weakness in the gut muscle.

Nutritional and lifestyle advice contained in the last two parts of this book should help you alleviate the problem of straining and constipation.

Ribbon stools, painful to pass

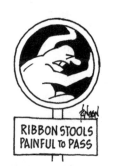

RIBBON STOOLS PAINFUL To PASS

If your bowel movements look ribbon-like, it means that your bowel is spastic, and that the mucous coating of your bowel is inflamed or dried out. Almost certainly, some sections of your bowel are swollen. As the stool can't pass out easily, it comes out as a ribbon, trying to make its way through the sections of the bowel that are suffering from inflammation.

A 'sore bowel' is very much like a sore throat. If you think how difficult it can be to swallow when your throat is inflamed, imagine that the bowel lining is very similar to the throat lining.

However, it has fewer nerve endings that are part of the central nervous system, so it takes a while for the condition to build up and for you to take notice.

You can deal with this problem nutritionally. Try to eliminate spicy foods, carbonated drinks, alcohol and coffee from your diet.

Have 'warm, wet, boring meals': runny porridge, vegetable soups and stews with some grains, such as brown rice or barley, warm fruit compotes and jelly. Keep your meals small and do not sit down or bend down for about 20 minutes after each meal. Avoid anything that is too hot or too cold.

Diarrhoea

Diarrhoea is a defence mechanism. If you have diarrhoea, it means that you have consumed something that the bowel is trying to eliminate or that you have caught a bug.

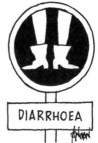

In order to help trigger the defecation process as quickly as possible, the bowel will not extract as much fluids out of the stools as it would do under healthy circumstances. This will enable the body to get rid of the offending substance and start the healing process.

If diarrhoea stops of its own accord after a day or two and gradually gets better, it means that the body has mobilized its immune defence potential.

Do not ignore diarrhoea

If diarrhoea starts wearing you down, you definitely need to think about supporting your body's healing potential with whatever means you are used to.

Some people prefer natural ways, which include extra hydration, taking large amounts of probiotics to stimulate bowel acidity and the fermentation process, increasing their intake of live yoghurt, taking mucilage herbs, such as slippery elm, using charcoal, etc. Others will go to the doctor, who may prescribe the relevant medication.

On the whole, diarrhoea is one way of the bowel telling you that the body needs support. Please don't ignore these signs. Give your body support when it needs it, and it will give you support when you need it.

Remember that constipation and diarrhoea could also be consequences of stress, taking antibiotics, going on holiday, increasing or decreasing your level of physical activity, and of any sudden or drastic changes that the body and the mind are not prepared for.

Blood in your stools

If you have fresh blood in your bowel, it might mean that your stool was too heavy and dry. It may have scratched the bowel wall, causing it to bleed. If blood continues to appear in your stools, you must seek medical advice.

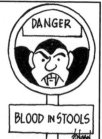

If you have darkened blood in your stools, this means that you have a haemorrhage somewhere higher up - possibly in your stomach or small intestine. Seek advice, and don't put off contacting your doctor. Make sure you undergo all the tests that are available to determine the source of dark blood.

Improving the quality of your eliminations

Part Four contains specific advice on how to improve your elimination through healthy living and exercise.

But there are other factors that come into play, and I think the whole story of successful eliminations would not be complete if I didn't mention them.

First of all, everyone needs to understand and accept that bowel cleansing is a natural process for us humans. It is a private thing, but it is not a dirty or shameful thing. Try to find an opportunity to open your bowels when they ask for it.

Be comfortable

When you go to the toilet, try to make yourself comfortable. In many countries, disposable toilet seat covers are now provided.

When you sit on the toilet, if you can raise your feet and put them on a small stools in front of you, this will be a great help to your bowel. This is how we are designed to evacuate: squatting over a hole in the ground, not sitting on a toilet.

Take time

The next important thing is to give yourself time to release fully. Modern life is not conducive to taking time out in the middle of the morning to sit on the toilet for 10 minutes, to make sure you have given your bowel sufficient time to complete its task.

However, if we can make time for a conversation with a colleague, a cigarette, a quick trip to a coffee shop, or for a chat or text over the mobile phone, we should also be able to make quality time to help the body with its eliminations.

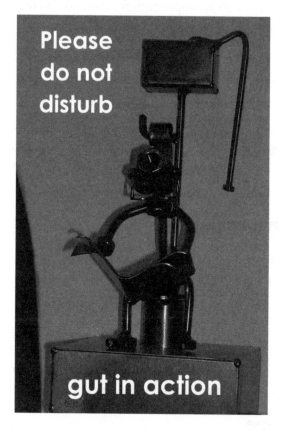

If you suffer from digestive complaints such as constipation, bloatedness or a heavy feeling after a meal, I would definitely recommend performing daily the bowel support and digestive health exercises described at the end of this book.

Respect your second brain

Generally, it is worth remembering that the bowel is our second brain. Treat your bowel in the same way as you would treat your brain: keep it active for some of the time, and then give it breaks, so that it can replenish its resources.

In the same way that you wouldn't want destructive and angry thoughts to rent too much space in your brain, you wouldn't want too many harmful and nutrient-depleted foods to take space in your bowel.

Summary: your road map to winning the poo

- The seven important bowel functions include:
  - massaging the organs of the abdominal cavity;
  - recycling water and nutrients back into circulation;
  - producing serotonin, our mood-regulating neuro-transmitter;
  - producing vitamin K and some vitamins of the B group;
  - producing stool-fermenting enzymes and fermenting wastes;
  - supporting the body's immune system;
  - eliminating digestive wastes.
- The large intestine is a sealed ecosystem that accommodates between 200 and 500 different colonies of bacteria. Dangers to this ecosystem come from our food and lifestyle choices: excessive sugar, alcohol, cigarettes, antibiotics, painkillers and processed foods are some of the greatest enemies of beneficial bacteria.
- It isn't unreasonable to eliminate somewhere in the

region of 200g of faeces a day, for a food intake of about 2 kg, and more if we eat more.

- If you have a reasonably established pattern, and have a feeling that nothing is left in the lower gut and you feel lighter and relieved after getting off the toilet, it means your digestive system is doing its job.

- If you feel heavy and bloated and, even when you go daily, you don't feel relieved, it means your digestive system isn't working as efficiently as it could be.

- The quality of your eliminations can tell you a lot about your digestive system.

- Treat your bowel in the same way as you would treat your brain: keep it active, but give it breaks to replenish its resources.

- Give your bowel the support that it deserves, and it will provide you with support when you need it.

Test Your Knowledge

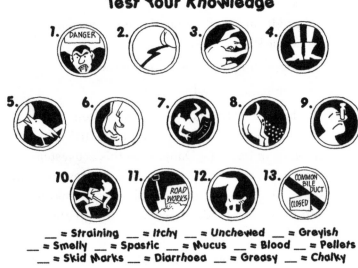

__ = Straining __ = Itchy __ = Unchewed __ = Greyish
__ = Smelly __ = Spastic __ = Mucus __ = Blood __ = Pellets
__ = Skid Marks __ = Diarrhoea __ = Greasy __ = Chalky

Part Four

HEALTHY DIGESTION AND WEIGHT MANAGEMENT

KEEP YOURSELF LIGHT

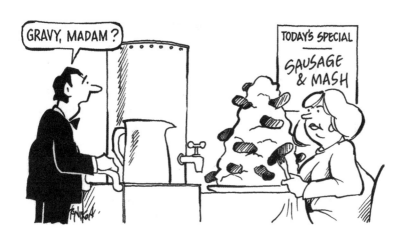

PART FOUR: HEALTHY DIGESTION AND WEIGHT MANAGEMENT

Seven rules of healthy digestion and weight management

- Chew properly

- Eat naturally hard foods

- Know when you are full

- Eat for what you are about to do, not what you have done

- Keep your meals simple, and don't mix too many different types of foods in one meal

- Keep your meals mostly alkaline, by volume

- Buy locally and buy in season

Summary: your road map to healthy digestion and weight management

Seven rules of healthy digestion and weight management

SEVEN RULES OF HEALTHY DIGESTION AND WEIGHT MANAGEMENT

1. Chew properly.

2. Eat naturally hard foods.

3. Know when you are full.

4. Eat for what you are about to do, not what you have done.

5. Keep your meals simple, and don't mix too many different types of foods in one meal.

6. Keep your meals mostly alkaline, by volume.

7. Buy locally and buy in season.

The wide-angled view

It amuses me that carnivores hunt for their food and devour it while it is fresh and juicy; herbivores chew their food to distraction.

Man, as an omnivore, sits in the middle, so your safe bet is to go with herbivores when eating carbohydrates, and you won't get it wrong.

Let us take a wide-angled snapshot of our digestion and get a general view of what is going on.

Our digestive system, i.e. the 'complicated tube' between our mouth and anus, is about four to five times as long as we

---

are tall. We only have voluntary control over the first part of the system, which is our mouth, and the last part of the system, which is our anus.

These are the only two sections of the digestive system that are monitored by our head brain through the central nervous system. It means that we can consciously decide whether we are going to open our mouth to put food into it, how we are going to chew and when we are going to swallow. Also, we can consciously open our bowels to eliminate wastes.

Chew properly

Therefore, chewing is the key to the rest of your digestive system, and this is one of the crucial factors that will affect the quality of your evacuations.

Chewing properly is beneficial for a number of reasons.

CHEW PROPERLY

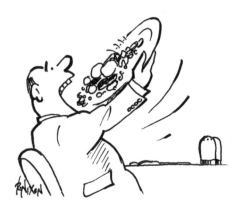

- Saliva moistens the food. It contains the digestive enzyme amylase, which starts breaking down long chains of complex carbohydrates, helping the rest of the digestive system to turn them into simple sugars and use them for energy.

- Chewing also warms up and moistens proteins and fats, thus preparing them for processing by the stomach acid and other digestive enzymes in the small intestine.

- Saliva is also a mild antiseptic that destroys some of the undesirable microbes present in our food.

- By chewing slowly, we 'unlock' the taste of the food and learn to appreciate it more.

- When we take time to unlock the taste of food in the mouth, the head brain gets the message and gives the mouth the command to swallow. In this scenario, it is easier for the brain to understand when we are full, and recommend us to stop eating.

> If you watch slim people in restaurants, they have a common pattern of eating: they chew slowly, and then put the fork down.
>
> Then they pick up the fork, carefully arrange the food on it, put the food in their mouth, chew it, put the fork down again, have a chat with their companion, and then take another mouthful of their food.
>
> It takes them quite a while to eat their food, and a lot of the time they are quite happy to leave on the plate even the things they like. That is a very good habit to acquire.

- Chewing slowly is the cheapest and safest method of weight management: spend your time chewing properly for a week or two and see how much less you need to eat.

Stop gassing

Another good habit is to keep your mouth shut while you are chewing. It is not only quite a civilized thing to do, but it also stops air bubbles getting into the digestive system.

The digestive system will generate enough of its own air bubbles in the process of food fermentation, so you really don't need to get more air into your gut before it starts generating its own gas. Air that comes into the digestive system with food can contribute to bloatedness and discomfort.

Eat naturally hard foods

There must be a reason why we have a mouth full of very strong teeth, the hardest substances in the body. The reason is that we are designed to chew, or masticate, hard foods.

Whole foods - pulses, such as beans and peas, and grains such as rice, barley, oats, buckwheat, quinoa, and millet - are naturally hard foods. So are many uncooked nuts, seeds, fruit and root vegetables.

Hard foods are full of fibre

Hard foods contain nutrients in the most natural form; they are nutritionally dense and rich. They also contain fibre, or roughage - nature's favourite bowel brush.

Grains contain soluble fibre that helps bulk up the stools and retain moisture in them. Vegetables and pulses contain soluble and insoluble fibre; insoluble fibre ferments in the large intestine, making the stools bulky and heavy, and prevents the formation of plaque on the bowel wall.

Eating naturally hard food keeps our teeth and gums healthy and can prevent gum diseases.

Eating hard food is your insurance policy

The best policy is to have naturally hard foods, high in fibre, in your diet, if you wish to have a healthy digestive system, and use foods as prevention against degenerative diseases.

Soaking beans, pulses and grains overnight and discarding the soak water awakens the grain and reduces cooking time. If you eat them slightly undercooked - al dente, Italian style - then you can guarantee that you will develop a proper chewing habit very quickly.

All naturally hard foods require chewing to unlock their taste, and, as you already know, the more we chew, the better

EAT NATURALLY HARD FOODS

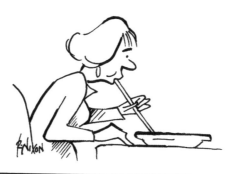

we digest and the less we eat - the ultimate win-win situation.

Eating hard foods is your best protection against overeating. If you have to chew the food, and its hidden taste is not obvious the moment you put it in your mouth, you have to make more effort to break the starchy chains.

Help your digestion by eating less and establishing a better connection between your mouth, your brain and your stomach, so you have a true feeling of fullness.

Be vigilant when eating soft foods

This is why I strongly advise my clients against eating soft foods with sauces, such as pastas, curries and kormas: the brain perceives the taste the moment you put these foods into your mouth, you swallow and go for the next forkful straight away. By the time your gut tells you that you have had enough, you have definitely eaten too much.

Beans and pulses

Beans are a very healthy food: about 80% of the nutrition in some cultures comes from beans, and these are the cultures with the strongest digestive systems.

If you are not used to eating beans and pulses, introduce them into your diet very carefully. Start by adding two or three spoonfuls of beans, which you have soaked and slightly undercooked, to your salads, steamed or grilled dishes and stews.

You need to make that sure your gut adjusts to the fibre in the beans and is allowed time for strong and robust fibre-fermenting bacteria to settle in and get ready for some good work.

Little by little, you can gradually start adding more fibre. You could even begin sprouting pulses and beans, such as mung beans, chickpeas etc., and grains, such as wheat berries. Sprouted beans and grains are probably amongst the most nutritious and cheapest foods available to us.

Know when you are full

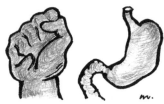

The stomach is roughly the size of your fist

Keeping yourself light is all about knowing when to stop eating, and it makes a lot of common sense.

If we go back to the similarities between the bowel and the brain, you will see very clearly that both need to rest in order to recharge themselves.

Keeping your body light, not overeating and controlling your appetite have historically been virtues in many religious and personal development systems.

One of the maxims popular in Eastern philosophies states that after a meal your stomach should be one-third solid foods (on the bottom), one-third liquids (in the middle), and one-third 'sacred fire', or spirit (on top).

If in 20 minutes' time after finishing your meal you are still hungry, it means that you have not had enough. It always takes the brain around 20 minutes to register that you are full.

A good thing to remember every time you eat is that your stomach is roughly the size of your clenched fist - it is not that big at all!

In Europe, when nannies were bringing up the children of aristocrats in the nineteenth century, they always told them that the golden rule of good digestion is: leave the table feeling slightly hungry, and wait for at least 20 minutes before asking for more.

This golden rule should especially apply to those who have a tendency to 'suck in' their food too quickly.

Eating too quickly equals eating too much

When you eat quickly, and especially when you don't chew your food properly, the food drops down the oesophagus into the stomach and then into the small intestine, and it is only when it starts backing up from the small intestine into the

KEEP YOURSELF LIGHT

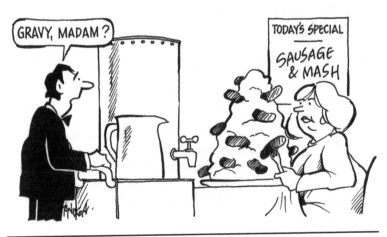

stomach that you realize you've had enough.

By this time you have eaten too much and created a bottleneck in your stomach and small intestine, which it will take a while for the body to clear, and you will feel slightly heavy and lethargic after a meal.

One of the main reasons for this is that a lot of blood needs to be diverted to the stomach to do the clearout after your feast, and the brain does not get the oxygen that it needs to function properly, so it goes into its energy-saving mode.

Pick or pack?

There is a lot of debate about whether people should eat smaller meals and graze, or have a big sitting, with a proper meal, and gorge. Pick or pack?

Well, no two people are the same. For many people, especially women, having smaller meals throughout the day works quite well. On the other hand, there are others who prefer a full three course meal once a day and very little for the rest of the time.

Birds and cows pick, leopards and snakes pack. Try either picking of packing, and decide what is best for you.

Don't pick and pack

Don't do both though. What you shouldn't be doing is having three or more meals a day and overeating constantly, because you are then constantly asking your digestive system to work without any breaks, slave-driving it into an early grave.

Eat light under stress

Eat light when you are under stress. When you are in the middle of a 'fight-or-flight' situation, your heart is beating and your brain is focused on finding a way out. If you are running late for a meeting and need to finish your notes and so on, a lot of adrenalin gets pumped into the system.

This alone gives the digestive system the signal to shut down for a while to divert the blood to the other systems in the body, where oxygen is needed much more.

If in the middle of your stressful situation you sit down and have a huge meal, it is not going to make things any easier: it is not going to reduce the amount of adrenalin in your system.

What it is going to do is slow down digestion even further. When the digestion is slowed down the food starts to decompose before the body has had the chance to absorb the nutrients from it. Bloatedness and discomfort often originate from eating too much under stress.

Learn to read the messages

Your body naturally tends to keep itself light: don't override messages of satiety from your brain - it will stop giving them eventually, and your health will suffer as a result. In the same way, don't override messages to open your bowel. Keep yourself light by listening to both brains!

Eat for what you are about to do, not what you have done

We all know that in order to have a balanced intake of nutrients we need carbohydrates and fibre, proteins and fats, vitamins and minerals.

Carbohydrates are mostly used for energy, proteins for rebuilding the cells, and fats for enabling chemical processes in the body, for optimal brain function and for long-term energy storage.

There are different theories about how best to balance fats, proteins and carbohydrates during the day: there are as many theories as there are authors.

Some researchers think we should have 80% carbohydrates, 10% proteins and 10% fats, others believe that we need carbohydrates, proteins and fats in roughly equal proportions.

So, how are you going to find out what is good for you?

Consider your lifestyle

Imagine your day as a series of events, each of which places different demands on different functions of your body.

Take the morning, for example.

When we get up, some of us have a workout that engages the muscles and the respiratory system. Others prepare children for school, which requires a multi-tasking ability, good memory and emotional stability.

Others go straight to their computer, to do some mental work, and don't get away till lunchtime. Others drive 30-40 miles to an important meeting, trying to negotiate traffic, prepare for closing their deal, and try to keep stress levels down.

And then there are some who have just come back from the night shift or a long-haul flight, and they go straight to bed.

Irrespective of what we are about to do, we also need to get our digestion going and to keep ourselves hydrated.

In addition to this, some of us are morning people, and some are night people. Some are driven by carbohydrates; some need more proteins to help regulate their blood sugar and energy flow.

Our nutritional demands are different

So our nutritional demands in the morning will be different, because everyone is unique and we all start the day differently.

The same happens throughout the day. Some of us work sitting in front of the computer engaging the head brain, or doing some repetitive tasks that require attention to detail.

Some are engaged in physical work all day. Some work shifts, and so on. Some of us are pickers, some are packers. We are all genetically unique - no two people are the same.

Therefore, I am convinced that the best way to find your ideal diet is to identify the demands that your lifestyle places on your body, and tailor your nutritional choices to meeting these demands.

Maximize nutritious foods

Remember that all the tasks you undertake during the day need to be supported by nutrient-rich and enzyme-rich food. So, as a general rule, maximize fresh, living foods and minimize foods full of 'empty calories', such as processed foods, sodas, simple sugars and alcohol drinks.

EAT FOR WHAT YOU ARE ABOUT TO DO, NOT FOR WHAT YOU HAVE DONE

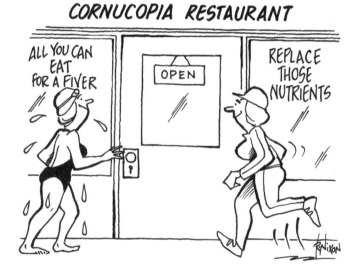

The basic rules

• If you are about to engage in medium-level physical activities, eat some slow-burning carbohydrates, which are great for a steady influx of energy. A soup or stew containing vegetables, rice or barley is a good example of an energy-saving meal.

- An injection of high-energy carbohydrates (such as a fresh fruit juice) and slow-burning carbohydrates (such as wholemeal pitta with a filling of your choice) would be great before a short burst of any serious physical activity, such as a training session.

- Do not eat immediately before training - you gut is the one muscle that does not need exercising during your work-out!

- Do not have a heavy meal after a workout just because you have expended energy - replenish your reserves with small quantities of nutrient-rich food. Fresh, living foods are the best after a workout, and your body will appreciate the enzymes and easy-to-assimilate nutrients.

- If you know that you will not be able to have another meal for a while, make sure your 'pre-event' snack or meal contains proteins and carbohydrates, because proteins slow down carbohydrate digestion, allowing you to 'stretch' the filling effect of your meal. A jacket potato with tuna fish filling and a salad should last you quite a while.

- If you need to resolve a mental challenge, a fresh fruit

> **If you are about to expend energy over and above your life support needs (breathing, moderate movement, mental tasks and digestion), make sure you have given your body a source of extra energy. However, if you are not doing anything special, your calorie intake should be sufficient for, but not above, those needs.**

salad or fruit juice would be great, because you will need the glucose, with a few seeds and nuts thrown in to 'oil the cogs' in your brain. Another good mental energy support is a fresh fruit smoothie with live yoghurt.

- Fibre is something we need throughout the day to maintain good elimination - eat high-fibre snacks, such as fresh and dry fruit, berries and vegetables.

- Water is required to keep us hydrated - drink water throughout the day.

- Your last meal of the day should be rich in vegetables and proteins, which your body will use for re-building the cells at night.

- Go to bed on an empty stomach (stop eating at least 2 ½ to 3 hours before bedtime).

- Your intake of nutrients - vitamins, minerals and enzymes - should always be high.

Keep your meals simple, and don't mix too many different types of foods in one meal

Keep it simple

The golden rule of achieving any visible changes in your lifestyle is keeping it simple.

If you want to exercise, don't wait for an opportunity to go to a posh gym; walk every day and/or do some rebounding instead.

If you want to get rid of cellulite, drink a lot of water, exercise, eat lots of vegetables and fruit and use a dry skin

KEEP YOUR MEALS SIMPLE AND DON'T MIX TOO MANY DIFFERENT TYPES

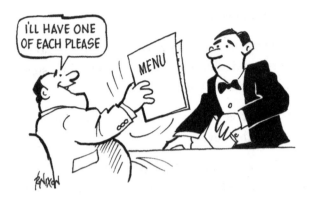

brush daily. This will make more sense on a day-to-day basis than going for expensive treatments.

The same thing applies to your meals: keep them simple.

Imagine a typical three-course meal: salmon and salad for a starter, then some red meat and vegetables or potatoes for your main course and a chocolate cake for dessert - plus a couple of glasses of wine, a helping of olives and so on.

In effect, you are asking the body to do quite a few things simultaneously: to digest slow-burning carbohydrates and fibre (your salad and vegetables), fast-burning carbohydrates, alcohol and glucose (potatoes, wine and cake) and two different kinds of animal proteins (fish and meat), all of which you have all ingested in the space of an hour.

Could you be asking too much? It is obvious that the body won't be able to digest it all at once, so don't be surprised if you feel heavy, bloated and tired after a meal like this.

So, here is my advice on how to keep it simple:

The rules of keeping it simple

- Eat when you are hungry, not because food is there.

- If you feel you want to eat something, such as a salad, soup, baked potato or yoghurt, eat that one thing only. Do not turn it into a three-course meal just because you have sat down at the table.

- Keep your fridge and cupboard lean: do not buy too many different foods just because they look good, they are on a special deal, or even if they are good for you.

- Be a conscious shopper and eater: buy and eat small amounts of high-quality fresh food.

- Clear your fridge of old food once a week, and see how much you have wasted.

- Buy less.

- When eating out remember that most of the time you

Emotional eating, i.e. eating anything in sight as a form of guilt management when you are bored, insecure, disappointed, fed up or let down, will make you feel more bored, insecure, disappointed, fed up or let down. It will also make you constipated, bloated, sick and overweight.

If you are an emotional eater, re-write this sentence on a large piece of paper and put it on your fridge door.

---

do not need more than two courses to satisfy your nutritional needs.

- If you are invited to a barbeque or an 'eat as much as you want' meal, remember that most of the time it is

KEEP YOUR MEALS MOSTLY ALKALINE BY VOLUME

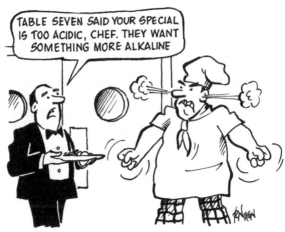

TABLE SEVEN SAID YOUR SPECIAL IS TOO ACIDIC, CHEF. THEY WANT SOMETHING MORE ALKALINE

also a great opportunity for catching up, socializing and networking, for both your personal and business needs. Put these needs first, and you will not feel as hungry.

- Use simple food-combining rules to make digestion easier: animal proteins combine with vegetables; grains and potatoes combine with vegetables. Fruits are better eaten on their own. Processed foods are better left out altogether.

- Sometimes you are not hungry, you are just thirsty. Drink some water first.

Remember that if you have taken control of this part of your life, you will be able to regain control of other parts of your life.

Keep your meals mostly alkaline, by volume

You would have heard of pH balance: 'p' stands for 'potential, and 'H' stands for hydrogen. Body pH measures the number of hydrogen ions in solution in body fluids.

Body pH is measured on the scale of 0 to 14. Anything less than 6.4 is considered to be acidic, anything over 6.4 is alkaline.

The human body is generally an alkaline environment. Blood maintains its pH at 7.3, saliva and urine should be around 6.4 if you eat and live healthily.

The one exception to the 'alkaline equals healthy' law is the digestive system, especially the stomach and the intestines that have to fight undesirable bacteria and micro-organisms. This is probably one of the reasons why they are acidic, bug-zapping, environments. The stomach pH can be as low as 2, and that of the intestines about 4 (out of 14).

Alkaline and acidic ash

All foods form a residue in the body, called ash. This residue can be either acidic or alkaline in nature. Most fruits and vegetables, as well as sprouted seeds, nuts, grains and pulses, form an alkaline ash when fully assimilated.

All animal products, including milk, cheeses and yoghurts, all processed foods and unsprouted grains, seeds, nuts and pulses form an acidic ash when fully assimilated.

Acidity and alkalinity are quite complicated subjects, but, to put it in very simple terms, between 70% and 80% of what we eat should be alkaline and between 20% and 30% of what we eat should be acidic.

Things can be alkaline, even if they taste acidic. Most fruit and vegetables are alkaline, even lemons and oranges. Although they don't taste sour, eggs, cheese, fish, white meat, and read meat are acidic, as are most grains.

If you keep your meals mainly alkaline by volume, you will help your body maintain an optimum pH balance.

Practical tips

In practice, keeping meals alkaline means that whenever you sit down to have a meal, you should make sure that half of your plate is taken up by vegetables or salads and the other half is divided into two - one of the quarters being taken up by grains and the remaining quarter by proteins.

If you eat lots of grains, such as brown rice, buckwheat, barley, wheat berries and rye, the way to make them more alkaline is to soak them overnight and discard the soak water. The same applies to seeds, nuts, beans and pulses. As you awaken the germ in the grain, it starts to become more alkaline.

Make sure you chew well to increase the alkalinity of starches.

Buy locally and buy in season

By purchasing your groceries from local farm shops and local farmers' markets, you will always get nutrient-rich, fresh

Examples of acid-forming foods

Proteins
- Bacon
- Beef
- Carp
- Clams
- Cod
- Corned Beef
- Fish
- Haddock
- Lamb
- Lobster
- Mussels
- Organ Meats
- Oyster
- Pike
- Pork
- Rabbit
- Salmon
- Sardines
- Sausage
- Scallops
- Shellfish
- Shrimp
- Tuna
- Turkey
- Veal
- Venison

Most Grains
- Amaranth
- Barley
- Bran, oat
- Bran, wheat
- Bread
- Corn
- Cornstarch
- Crackers, soda
- Flour, wheat
- Flour, white
- Hemp Seed Flour
- Kamut
- Macaroni
- Noodles
- Oatmeal
- Oats (rolled)
- Quinoa
- Rice (all)
- Rice Cakes
- Rye
- Spaghetti
- Spelt
- Wheat Germ
- Wheat

Poultry
Eggs
Refined Sugars
Food Additives

Most Dairy, such as Butter, Cheese & Yoghurt

Examples of alkalizing foods

Vegetables
- Alfalfa
- Barley Grass
- Beet Greens
- Beets
- Broccoli
- Cabbage
- Carrot
- Cauliflower
- Celery
- Chard Greens
- Chlorella
- Collard Greens
- Cucumber
- Eggplant
- Fermented Veggies
- Garlic
- Greens and Beans
- Kale
- Lettuce
- Mushrooms
- Onions
- Parsnips
- Peas
- Peppers
- Pumpkin
- Radishes
- Sea Veggie
- Spinach, Green
- Sprouts
- Sweet Potatoes
- Tomatoes
- Watercress
- Wheat Grass

Fruits
- Apple
- Apricot
- Avocado
- Banana
- Berries
- Cantaloupe
- Cherries, sour
- Coconut, fresh
- Currants
- Grapes
- Grapefruit
- Lemon
- Lime
- Melon
- Nectarine
- Orange
- Peach
- Pear
- Pineapple
- Raisins
- Rhubarb
- Tangerine
- Tropical Fruits
- Watermelon

BUY LOCAL AND BUY IN SEASON

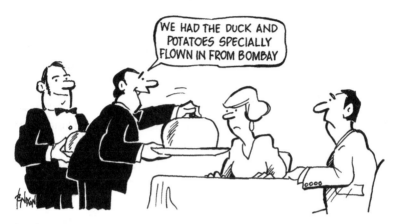

food, and you will contribute to the survival of organic farming in your area.

Organic foods

Many people ask me whether they should eat organic foods. My answer to this is: yes, it makes sense to eat organic, if organic is also local. Any fresh food organically farmed a few thousand miles away would be a lot less organic by the time it got to the supermarket, and even less so by the time it got on your plate.

Become a seasonal eater

Also, if you live in a country that has seasons, eating in season is something your digestive system would probably appreciate. Eat light; make sure you have plenty of fresh, uncooked food in the warm and hot season. During the hot season, eat in the morning and in the evening, when it is cooler.

As the cold season and winter set in, you may feel the need to have slightly heavier, warmer meals, preserved foods etc.

Eat short-life fruits and vegetables in season: pick your own raspberries, strawberries, plums and asparagus and eat them fresh while they are at the peak of their nutrient value.

Be an educated shopper

Turn shopping into a fun pastime for yourself and your family: go to the farmers' market and make sure you ask the farmers how they grow their food and where it comes from. Make a trip to the farmers' market a colour-rich, emotionally uplifting and intellectually rewarding day out for the whole family.

Growing bean and seed sprouts is a healthy and inexpensive way of getting fresh food all year round.

Educate yourself about edible wild-growing herbs, berries and mushroom in your area, and go picking with your children, then cook and eat the food that you have yourselves harvested. These simple things will help you understand the nutritional and emotional value of nourishing foods.

The eighty-twenty rule

Remember one simple thing: you are eating most of the time for nourishment, and some of the time for pleasure. So when you eat for nourishment, do what you need to do to keep your body happy; don't overtax it and don't give it too much stuff that it won't appreciate.

Sometimes, on occasion, you eat just for pleasure! When you do, choose what you want, what your mind wants, what your senses want, what your feeling of satisfaction wants, but keep it all in proportion: 80% good and 20% letting your hair down.

Whatever you do, make sure you enjoy it, and you don't make your body suffer for it.

Summary: your guide to healthy digestion and weight management

Healthy eating and weight management only works if you follow a system of rules. Any system you develop must reflect your unique circumstances and lifestyle requirements. Whatever system you create for yourself, it will make a lot of common sense to incorporate the rules below.

- Chew properly: proper chewing is an essential part of healthy digestion. It is probably the cheapest and the most reliable form of weight management. Good chewing is one of the best remedies against bloatedness, gassiness, heavy feeling after a meal or overeating.

- Eat naturally hard foods, such as grains, seeds, nuts, beans, pulses and vegetables. Naturally hard foods are usually nutrient-rich and calorie-poor. Eating hard foods that are high in fibre is your insurance policy against degenerative diseases and your best protection against overeating. Eating foods al dente, or slightly undercooked, will also help proper chewing and better digestion.

- Know when you are full: your body naturally tends to keep itself light. Don't override messages of satiety from your brain - it will stop giving them eventually, and your health will suffer as a result. Eat light when you are under stress.

- Choose whether you should 'pick' or 'pack', but don't do both!

- Eat for what you are about to do, not what you have done. Make sure your food intake reflects the demands of your lifestyle. Eating should reflect your future needs, rather than past efforts. This means, for example, that eating a fuller meal in the morning, before the day's events, makes more sense that eating a big dinner after the event.

- Keep your meals simple, and don't mix too many different types of foods in one meal, Become a conscious eater and a conscious shopper: buy and eat small amounts of high-quality fresh food.

- Keep your meals mostly alkaline, by volume. Human physiology is better adjusted to digesting alkaline foods. In practice, keeping meals alkaline means that whenever you sit down to have a meal, you should make sure that half of your plate is taken up by vegetables or salads, whilst the other half is divided into two - one of the quarters being taken up by grains and the other quarter by proteins.

- Buy locally and buy in season. By purchasing your groceries from local farm shops and local farmers' markets, you will always get nutrient-rich, fresh food, and you will contribute to the survival of organic farming in your own country.

PART FIVE

SEVEN PILLARS OF HEALTHY LIVING

MAKE SURE YOU HAVE DAILY BOWEL MOVEMENTS.....

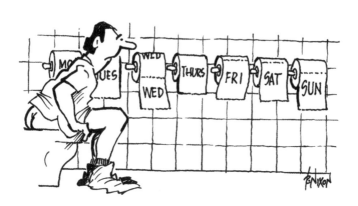

PART FIVE:
SEVEN PILLARS OF HEALTHY LIVING

Breathe and let breathe

Hydrate your body

Nourish your emotions

Lymphasize

Exercise

Eat living foods

Cleanse

Summary: your road map to healthy living

Let us take a step back

At the initial stages of human development, food was used largely for nourishment, and occasionally as a gift. In our modern life, food has changed its role quite significantly.

Ancient Greeks assigned food a new role - that of entertainment and status symbol. Epicureans derived great pleasure from obscenely opulent meals.

As family units developed, food and family meals came to symbolize comfort, security and stability of life.

Food has lost its roots

Today food per se has come to be viewed as a disposable necessity, very much in the same way as some other attributes of our physiological existence, like a sanitary towel or a condom.

There is a whole generation of children who have been brought up on ready meals in plastic trays and who don't realize that food can actually be cooked in the kitchen from scratch, let alone be picked in a field and brought home.

I regularly encounter adult, university-educated, clients who don't know how to make a soup or how to boil rice, and who don't realize that bread and pasta were grains before they became bread and pasta.

Somehow in the food chain the connection between harvesting grains, growing vegetables and fruit and rearing animals, and ready-made meal that consist of barely identifiable components of all three has been lost.

You are judged by what you eat

On the other hand, diversity and availability of food in the Western world have brought choices, and it is fascinating how people can now be judged and labelled on the basis of the food choices that they make.

Those who eat natural foods and pay attention to where their food comes from are considered by society to be thoughtful and caring people. They are also considered to be trustworthy, thorough and progressive.

If someone is a vegetarian, or eats only organic food, then even before you know anything else about that person, you would probably have an image in your mind of someone who is responsible, reliable, honest and very slightly boring.

If someone eats sushi, that person is assumed to be a sophisticated trendy cosmopolitan living in a major city.

On the other hand, if you mention 'a burger and a cola a day man', it definitely conjures up the image of someone overweight, who is heading for heart disease, who obviously doesn't care about health and is digging his grave with his teeth.

Your gut is your judge

Whether we like it or not, we will be judged on the basis of our food choices - both by our peers and by our own digestive system. Even if you don't care about the opinion of your peers, the opinion of your digestive system determines to a great extent your health and quality of life, so it is definitely worth listening to it.

I hope I have convinced you that your gut is a creature of

habit. It likes organization, predictability and security. Making sure that it is happy does not take a lot, but it does require a system. So let us quickly look at some of the best-known systems.

Visual hooks for healthy eating

When you start looking after yourself in a meaningful way - watching what you eat, having respect for your digestion, doing some bodywork, colonics, emotional release treatments and so on - you start wondering what system you should adopt for yourself.

How can you introduce healthy changes into your lifestyle on a daily basis? How can you achieve a balance between enhanced quality of life and having fun, without turning your health into an obsession?

There are obviously a lot of systems on which you can base your own style and there are many hundreds of books on the market offering guidance on these systems.

Probably one of the easiest ways to create a usable system is to use a visual hook, an image that helps you remember your priorities. Different visual hooks work for different people.

The Food Pyramid

The best-known visual hook worldwide is a nutritional system called the food pyramid, which was first developed for the US Department of Agriculture:

The food pyramid is based on carbohydrates, particularly starches, as a foundation of good nutrition. As the pyramid

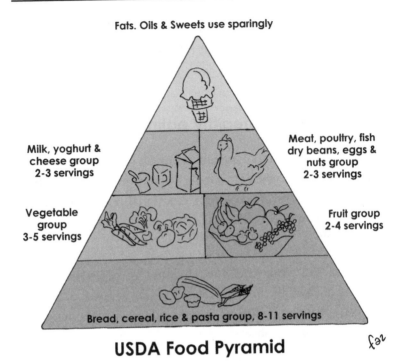

Fats. Oils & Sweets use sparingly

Milk, yoghurt & cheese group 2-3 servings

Meat, poultry, fish dry beans, eggs & nuts group 2-3 servings

Vegetable group 3-5 servings

Fruit group 2-4 servings

Bread, cereal, rice & pasta group, 8-11 servings

USDA Food Pyramid

narrows towards the tip, we see the proteins, fats, sweets and chocolates on top.

This is a good general guideline for someone who is just starting to review their nutritional choices. It has alerted many people to the importance of eating fruit and vegetables every single day.

The only serious problem with the food pyramid, in my view, is that all sweets and chocolates are at the top. We humans always take our bearings from the highest point, not from the lowest point. So it is not very good as a visual hook, because it may create a wrong image, making it harder to focus on the foundation of the pyramid, which is the grains, vegetables and fruit.

Food combining

Another very popular nutritional system is food combining.

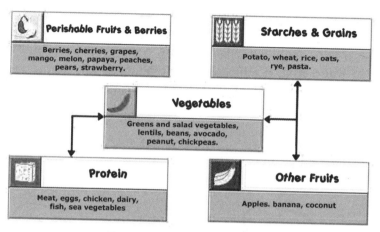

Food Combining

The food combining system is based on the different speeds of digestion of starches, vegetables, fruit and proteins.

Food combining, which should really be called 'food separating', involves separating heavy starches, such as potatoes or grains or pastas, from concentrated proteins such as meat, chicken or fish. A typical example of a 'wrong meal' in this system would be a roast dinner.

Supporters of food combining say that as it takes different lengths of time for nutrients to be digested, it makes sense to combine foods with roughly equivalent digestion times.

Therefore, you should eat beans and grains with vegetables, vegetables with proteins, and fruit on its own. Some people go to even greater lengths, by defining which fruits or vegetables you can eat with other fruit and vegetables and which ones would upset your digestion if you were to combine them.

This is a great system for a perfectionist, because it can be refined indefinitely.

I think that the food combining system is really useful in two ways: first, it educates people about food groups, and secondly, it makes their meals less heavy and rich in calories.

THE FOOD PYRAMID.....

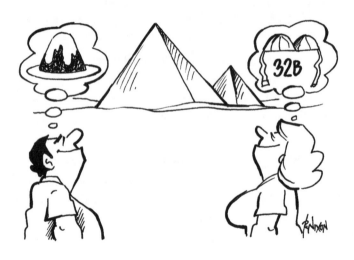

SEVEN PILLARS OF HEALTHY LIVING

I believe that food, although important, is only a small part of who we are. A couple of years ago, I started thinking about a visual hook that would work for me. When I came up with one, and shared it with my friends and colleagues, they started using it too.

They said it was easy to understand, useful and balanced, and suggested that I should share it with more people. So, here is my visual hook:

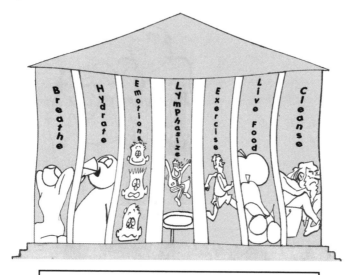

THE SEVEN PILLARS OF HEALTHY LIVING
1. **Breathe and let breathe.**
2. **Hydrate your body.**
3. **Nourish your emotions.**
4. **Lymphasize.**
5. **Exercise.**
6. **Eat living foods.**
7. **Cleanse.**

Breathe and let breathe

Breathing is the engine of life. We can live for a while without food and water, indefinitely without books, friends, clothes, café latte and sushi, but as soon as we stop breathing, we die. Breathing is also probably the most undervalued resource of health maintenance.

BREATHE AND LET BREATHE.....

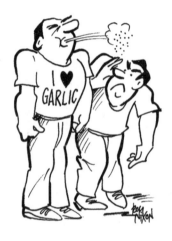

On average, we take over 15,000 breaths each day during our waking hours. Every one of them supports life in a direct and straightforward way.

There are a lot of resources related to breath work and proper breathing.

You learn different breathing systems when you do yoga, qui-gong or tai-chi exercises. You may have been introduced to various breathing systems if you have ever come across

Buteyko breathing, which is an extremely effective method of asthma management, or if you have been to any personal development courses or seminars, or if you have ever run or jogged.

Breathing tips

Here are the tips that you may find useful, on a day-to-day basis.

Watch your breath and listen to it. Close your eyes and silence your mouth for a few minutes, and listen to the flow of your breath, watching with your mind something that is invisible and powerful at the same time. It is a great exercise to do for a couple of minutes a few times a day, to relieve stress and energize your whole body.

Exercise your lungs: consciously fill the upper, middle and lower lobes of your lungs with oxygen, and then release the air. Remember that your lungs also cradle and massage your heart. In times of stress, you can consciously use your breathing to help your heart slow down.

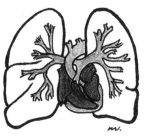

Use every opportunity to get fresh air. The air is much fresher and crispier early in the morning, which is the best time to go for a short brisk walk and set your body and mind for a healthy, rewarding day by nourishing them with oxygen.

Give your skin an airing

Remember that your skin, nails and hair also breathe. Unlike the internal organs, skin breathes independently from the lungs through direct oxygen exchange with the surrounding air. Skin breath is one of our most important detoxification pathways and body temperature regulators.

Make-up, acrylic nails and clothing made with man-made fibres such as nylon, stop the skin, the largest organ of your body, from breathing properly. Dress in natural fibres, remove make-up and let your hair down - use every opportunity to let your skin breathe, not only when you are on holiday, but at home too!

Hydrate your body

Hydration is something we all need. Our bodies are fluid. Our blood is our fluid connective tissue. Our lymph, which plays a crucial role in self-cleansing and protection from diseases and premature ageing, is also fluid. Our brains are mostly liquid. Reducing us to dry solids will leave us with almost nothing.

That is why it is crucially important to keep yourself hydrated. Questions are often asked about what we should drink. Obviously we can drink anything, because, at the end of the day, the body is sophisticated enough to try to draw water out of whatever it is given. Nevertheless, there are certain points that we need to remember

Limit sweet and carbonated drinks

Drinking sweet drinks is not the best way to hydrate your body, because sweet drinks contain sugar. Every unit of sugar requires nine units of water for processing, so by drinking sweet drinks you are giving your body just enough water to deal with the sugar that you have consumed in the same drink, with not much to spare.

Drinking carbonated drinks is not particularly harmful in itself, in moderation. However, if you do drink a lot of carbonated drinks, and especially those containing artificial sweeteners, they will leach calcium out of your bones and upset the balance of electrolytes in your digestive system, thus contributing not only to osteoporosis but also to bloatedness, heartburn and other digestive discomforts.

Drink water

Drinking water is probably the safest bet. Water is by far the best way to hydrate your body. You need to bear in mind that you are 70% water, so your intake of food and liquids throughout the day should contain at least 70% water.

Drink more water if you exercise, if it is warm or hot outside, if you are engaged in a physical activity, if you are on a detox or a fast, or if you are recovering from an illness or a stressful situation.

Drink the cleanest water you can find

Mineral water or tap water? Ideally, we should all live near a natural spring and drink great fresh mineral water, but for most of us this is not an option. So you can get bottled mineral water. When you do so, make sure that you know where it comes from, and that it has not been sitting in the sun in a plastic bottle. Also, change your brand of mineral water from time to time, to avoid overload of certain minerals and shortage of others.

The next best thing is to have a water filter to filter your tap water: let it run for the first 5 seconds and drink reasonably clean running water. It may not be 100% pure, but running water will be more oxygenated than still water from a plastic bottle, and oxygen is one of the most powerful bacteria-killing agents available.

The complexity of cleaning water reflects the complexity of modern life. Water companies are doing what they can to clean our water. There are certain things they can do, such as isolate known bacteria and solid wastes in the water or to filter the water in many different ways.

There are certain things water companies are unable to do well, and we should not blame them for this. They can't remove from the water all the antibiotics that we take and then excrete; they can't remove the hormonal wastes that are excreted by women on the pill and those on thyroxin for example.

In short: drink water, drink the cleanest water you can find, and drink enough of it to keep hydrated.

Nourish your emotions

Emotions and digestion

Emotions are such a big part of what we are. This is something I see a lot in my practice.

Sometimes people who come to me have a near-perfect diet, but their digestive systems do not work very well and they are not happy people.

There are other people, 'two burgers and a pint of lager a day' people, whose digestive systems actually work surprisingly well, especially considering what they put in.

One of the reasons why the digestive systems of some healthy eaters don't work, while some unhealthy eaters virtually get away with murder, is related to their different emotional make-ups and reactions to stress.

Happy people have good digestion

Happy, easy-going, emotionally balanced people can generally manage to stay cool in most situations of everyday life. They understand, or know intuitively, what they can change and what they can't, and they instinctively stay away from situations that they can not or choose not to change. They tend not to lose their temper very easily and they don't exaggerate the importance of little events.

Nevertheless, when they are confronted with a genuinely stressful situation, they can mobilize themselves, muster all the adrenalin they need and do what is required under pressure.

This balanced approach to life enables all their systems, including the digestive system, to work quite efficiently, even, for some, with the limited resources of their inadequate diets.

Unhappy people have digestion problems

Those of a more nervous disposition allow themselves to be influenced by a disproportionate rush of adrenalin, even after a minor event.

They get really wound up having to wait at a red light, or being obsessed with a deadline which in the real life doesn't mean anything. They can easily lose their confidence because of a conversation with a colleague who appears to be rude.

Those people who let small things shape their desperate attitude to life are actually quite unhealthy, despite any good diet that they might have. They are surviving rather than living.

They often suffer from constipation, water retention, IBS, heartburn, acid reflux, diarrhoea and other digestion problems, sometimes even on a good diet.

Put it all in prospective

There is no one way to stabilize and nourish our emotions, but here are some helpful hints:

The mind is a very powerful tool. If you let your mind race around chasing unfinished business, it will stress out every single cell of your body. You will be exhausted even before you get up in the morning! Every time you want to go into overdrive, ask yourself: 'Is whatever I am trying to chase up going to matter in 5 or 10 years' time?' Put it in prospective.

Events, positive and negative, occur daily. Things that you perceive as a personal offence are often not about you: someone being rude, forgetting about an appointment, giving you bad service etc, does not do it because of what you are. They do it because of what they are. You *choose to* be upset and to get worked up about the consequences. Again, remember: in most cases it is not about you.

Appreciate what you have got

Setting your mind on positive challenges is the same as asking every cell of your body to work effectively and efficiently, to stay young, to use nutrients in the best possible way, and to deliver the energy that will enable you to achieve your goals.

Nourish your emotion with the beauty around you, and cultivate beauty within you.

Appreciate what you have got, rather than getting worked up about what you have not got. If you have difficulty identifying the good things that you have got already, here is a short list you can use any time:

- Be grateful for the fact that you are living.

- Admire your ability to breathe the air, see the sun and touch the warm earth.

- You can travel, see the world, use Google, have food from all continents all year round, phone anyone in the world on your mobile phone and generally open yourself to growth every moment of your day.

Let us all remember that we are living in the amazing times, when anything is achievable if we put our mind to it!

You *choose to* be upset and to get worked up about the consequences of what you perceive as negative events. Again, remember: in most cases it is not about you!

Every time you want to go into overdrive, ask yourself: 'Is whatever I am trying to chase up going to matter in five or ten years' time?' Put it in perspective.

Lymphasize

Lymph is our cleansing fluid

Lymphasizing means activating the lymph. Lymph is a transparent fluid, a connective tissue that helps the body get rid of impurities and mount an effective immune defence against invaders. Our lymphatic system is designed as a cell-cleansing system: every single cell produces wastes, and these wastes get dumped into lymph.

Lymphatic nodes are the hubs of the lymphatic system: this is where the lymph is filtered after collecting cell wastes, and where bacteria and invaders are destroyed by lymphocytes.

It is interesting to know, for example, that white blood cells do not actually spend much time in the blood itself: they are stored in the bones and they are mostly released if and when they are required by the lymphatic system. They often use blood as a transportation route to get to the lymph nodes where they are needed.

Most lymphatic cells protect the gut

It is now thought that about 70% of all lymphatic cells may be located in our gut. One of the possible reasons for this is that the gut is the most vulnerable organ in our bodies.

The digestive system is an open-ended system, open at both ends, so it is not surprising that the mouth and the bowel are home to the largest colonies of bacteria. However, the mouth receives its dose of bacteria on the back of nutrients and oxygen, so on a good day it has a fair chance of getting the bacterial population under control. In addition, the entrance into the oesophagus is guarded by tonsils, which act as additional antibacterial lymphatic filters.

In the meantime, the bowel, as we know, gets very few nutrients, compared to other organs, but it does receive a lot of undesirable elements. That may be why there is such a huge colony of commensal and symbiotic bacteria, and why the bowel is home to about 70% of all the lymphatic cells. This is where the immune system has such an important role to play.

We need to activate the lymph

Whereas blood circulation is controlled by the heart, which pumps the blood around the body, the lymphatic system does not have its own pump. There are many ways to promote lymph renewal.

Practice deep breathing

The diaphragm, a dome-shaped sheet of muscle above our abdominal cavity, moves only 1 centimetre up or down in the course of shallow breathing, and up to 10 centimetres if we breathe deeply or during active exercise. This gently massages the lymph nodes in the abdominal cavity, helping move lymph around.

Dry skin brushing

One of the best ways to lymphasize is to do some dry skin brushing. Gentle dry skin brushing from the feet upwards, towards the heart, and down from the shoulders towards the heart accelerates the passage of lymph through the lymph nodes.

Contrast showering

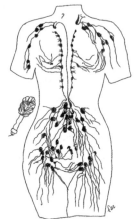

Dry skin brushing helps activate the lymphatic system

Another great method of pushing lymph round the body is to do contrast showering regularly. When you stand in the shower, try alternating warm and cold water. This increases blood circulation just below the skin surface and wakes up all the skin cells. Activity just below skin surface helps lymph vessels contract and relax, giving them the exercise they need. Also, it wakes you up, burns calories and reduces cellulite, gives you an adrenalin rush and decreases your appetite, all for the price of a simple shower.

Lymph drainage massage

Get a lymph drainage massage. Any massage will contribute to lymph drainage, but lymph drainage massage techniques have been developed specifically to address the challenges of the lymph renewal process. This is especially beneficial if you are on a detoxification or fasting programme.

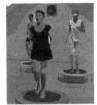

Rebounding also activates the lymphatic system.

Rebounding

Exercising is great for lymph renewal. One of the best forms of lymph drainage exercise is rebounding on a trampoline, which is often described as 'cellular exercise'. Rebounding activates the lymphatic system and cleanses all the body cells by flushing out metabolic wastes and saturating them with oxygen and enzymes. It is the only exercise that helps open and close the valves of the lymphatic vessels as you go up and down on the rebounder.

Vibration treatments

Vibration also works very well for lymphatic circulation. Vibration treatments are becoming more and more common: any automatic massage chair, which you can now find in airport lounges, major department stores and in health spas, as well as small portable devices, such as Chi machines, will give you a great lymphatic boost in 10-15 minutes.

Exercise

We are born to move, grow or catch our food, and expend a lot of energy simply to ensure our survival.

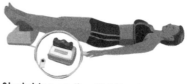

Stretching on the Chi Machine also activates the lymphatic system.

During our evolution, once we had acquired consciousness and the ability to make choices, our minds started 'moving' a lot more than our bodies, and we chose to go into a power-saving mode and move less. We need to remember though that our relative inactivity is a fairly recent phenomenon, in terms of human development.

We are programmed to move

Exercise, both mental and physical, is really important for good digestion. Every single cell of our body is programmed to move.

When I say 'exercise', I don't mean that you need to be a member of a gym or to work with a personal trainer, although if you enjoy gym work, it is a great way to build your health.

Exercise means movement: get up in the morning, spend about 5 or 10 minutes on a rebounder or a Chi machine, doing cellular exercise and awakening every single cell of your body. Later, go for a 20-minute walk during your lunch break, have a swim when you go to a spa, and do press-ups and abdominal exercises 5 days a week for 10 or 15 minutes per day, for example.

Exercise positively

Do something that you like doing: it could be aerobics, dance, yoga. The main thing is to do it because you love doing it and because you positively believe that it is going to enhance your quality of life. Every single cell of your body will enjoy this awakening, this call to be more active, to generate more energy, to absorb more nutrients and to stay younger for longer.

Exercise because you want to gain something, not lose something. Gain energy, gain youth, and gain an insight into how your body works. Don't do anything with a negative perspective, such as wanting to lose weight, or to burn without mercy all those calories that you have eaten. Negativity makes you acidic and, at the end of the day, unhealthy and often overweight.

Exercise your brain daily: make sure you resolve mental challenges; exercise your emotions, look at beauty every day, listen to great music, move your soul.

Exercise your physiology, smile, laugh or cry when you feel like it; you will find life a lot less stressful, and your bowel movements will improve.

Eat living foods

Now, finally, we come to nutrition. Where I come from, food is just one component of a much bigger picture, but a very important component.

There are as many nutritional systems and diets as there are nutritionists and diet specialists. Some good and some very good books on choosing your nutritional system are listed in below.

Remember that most of the time you eat for sustenance, but some time you eat for pleasure, comfort or joy. The foods that you choose for sustenance and for joy may be very different. Alcohol is hardly a life-sustaining nutrient, but sometimes a couple of glasses of good wine are exactly what your soul needs!

Sustainability

Whatever system you choose, make sure it is obtainable and sustainable. Yes, you can eat cabbage soup for a week, a month or even 2 months: the cabbage soup diet is certainly obtainable, but not sustainable.

At some point you will have to eat for pleasure and comfort, and your body and soul, deprived of comfort food for a couple of weeks or months, will consume every stodgy food within a two-mile radius.

Therefore in selecting a nutritional system you will need to see how expandable it is and whether it will be able to embrace different life situations: will it cope with you being sad, gutted, elated, failing an exam or dealing with a life-threatening disease?

Living foods

Like many optimists before me, and I suspect like many more optimists to come, I have spent a considerable amount of time developing a system that would be obtainable and sustainable. I think I have developed one. It works for me, and it works for my clients. It may or may not work for you, but try it first: EAT LIVING FOODS.

For some, it will be a fish fillet as opposed to fish fingers.
For some, it will be fresh food rather than frozen.
For some, it will be uncooked food rather than cooked.
For some, it will be organic rather than non-organic.
For some, it will mean going to a farm shop rather than a supermarket...

Living foods will be different for everyone, depending on their starting point:

Whatever living foods are for you, you need to step up your awareness of what you eat. Start where you are most comfortable, and move on from there.

Here, incidentally, is my version of the food pyramid.

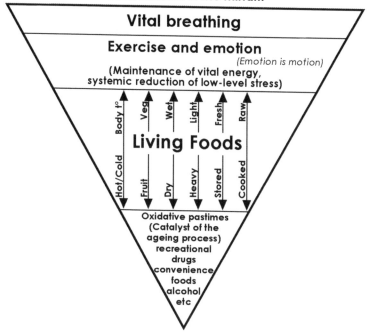

The Life-Food Balance
...the body is an outward, physical manifestation of the mind...

Vital breathing

Exercise and emotion
(Emotion is motion)
(Maintenance of vital energy, systemic reduction of low-level stress)

Living Foods

Body t° — Hot/Cold
Veg — Fruit
Wet — Dry
Light — Heavy
Fresh — Stored
Raw — Cooked

Oxidative pastimes (Catalyst of the ageing process) recreational drugs convenience foods alcohol etc

Food needs to have vital energy

I am a strong believer in eating foods that still have vital energy in them - the enzymes, the vitamins, the minerals and all other nutrients. Sometimes this vital energy is human: I will always choose a simple meal made with love and care by an illiterate cook in a poor eatery over a designer, pre-packaged macro-molecularly and nutritionally balanced ready meal from a supermarket.

The practice of eating living foods

Eat body temperature foods in preference to cold or hot foods

Body temperature foods are something that your body won't need to fight against. We all remember burnt tongues and peeling mucous lining of the mouth savaged by hot pizzas and curries, as well as teeth screaming after an ice-cream attack. One of the main reasons for spastic gut is drinking cold drinks in combination with hot food.

Choose vegetables first

I have enormous respect for fruit and vegetables, and particularly greens - they are nature's storehouses of vitamins and nutrients. Incidentally, I include sprouts in the vegetable category, to make it easier.

Vegetables are low-GI, high-bulk, high-fibre cleansing foods that, in my view, need to account for about at least 50% of anyone's food intake. They are varied and diverse both in taste and in texture, they are available all year round, they can be grown locally and they are within the price range of everyone.

Eat wet food rather than dry food

Wet food is, as a rule, more alive than dry food. Fresh food is, by definition, wet. Water brings life: soaked grains and nuts are more alive than non-soaked grains; a vegetable salad has more nutrients than a plate of French fries and so on.

Also, it is easier to eat wet food to help meet your fluid intake requirements. This is where fruits have a great role: an apple and a glass of water make more nutritional sense than a glass of water on its own.

Eat light foods in preference to heavy foods

Again, heavy foods tend to be stodgy and high in calories rather than nutrients. In winter, stodgy foods are comforting and warming, but in summer they place a heavy workload on the digestive system. As a general rule, make sure that you limit stodge and heavy sauces, and bulk up your meals with light, nutrient-rich vegetables and natural dressings.

Eat fresh food rather than stored food

I think this is a no-brainer, but a lot of people object to 'having to shop' too often to get fresh food. Well, it's your call: you would certainly turn down a defrosted cup of Cappuccino (yuk!) on aesthetic grounds - nothing short of a cup of coffee, freshly ground, and made in front of you, would be good enough.

By the same token, an omelette made with reconstituted egg powder, frozen ready meals and food quickly nuked in a microwave should have no place in your life, if you love yourself enough.

Eat raw rather than cooked

There is time and place for everything, and I think raw food should have a much more important place in our diet.

Eating raw means, for me, eating foods in the state in which they were grown or reared. There is a great variety in raw meals: I eat endless combinations of raw and fermented vegetables, salads, sprouts, fruit, nuts, cocoa beans, soya and fish, soaked seeds, shakes and so on; and of course, I drink fresh juices.

My rule of thumb

And finally, I'll share with you my rule of thumb when it comes to food: if you see something on your plate that you can't imagine having grown in a field or a garden, or having had a happy life, don't eat it! It won't do you any good...

Cleanse

Good nutrition, using bodywork, contrast showers, exfoliating, and obviously colon cleansing are very important, because if you are not achieving a good cleanse, it will mean that your cells are blocked up.

If the cells of your body are blocked up, they can't absorb nutrients; if they can't absorb nutrients, it is pointless having a good diet, and the vicious circle of ill-health will continue. Emotional blockages are just as detrimental as physical blockages: look at all those emotionally constipated people around you!

Today detoxing has become a very big issue. It is everywhere: on news stands, all over street advertisements, newspaper articles, TV commercials and posters in supermarkets.

Make the most of every day

There is a lot to be said for living a clean life. Being a monk in Tibet is different from being an options trader on Wall Street: the average life expectancy of a monk is close to 90 years, an average life of an options trader in Wall Street is probably a lot shorter.

However, very often it is about adding life to your years, rather than years to your life. There are very few people who would want to live to 200 years if it means spending many of them on a life support machine.

In this day and age, a lot is about here and now - how do

> **Yesterday is a history,**
> **tomorrow is a mystery,**
> **and today is a gift.**
> **This is why we call it**
> **'the present'.**

we make the most of the present? Remember the saying: 'Yesterday is a history, tomorrow is a mystery, and today is a gift: this is why we call it 'the present'.

A clean life is a rewarding life

It is not easy to live a clean life that is also a full, rewarding life, but it is certainly possible.

Here are some very simple, very general, pointers towards living a cleansed life, and they are not about food - they are about you.

- Do one thing every day that you find challenging, awkward or difficult. If you have control over a difficult, bothersome part of your life, it means that you have control over all other aspects of your life.

- Starting the day well can help you make good decisions for the rest of the day, and steer your life in the direction that it should take.

- Remember that every day counts and that time is the only thing you can't buy. Time is your greatest and most precious asset, and you should use it wisely.

- You can have generic computers, clothes or furniture. The only thing that can't be generic is your own life. If you feel you are getting sucked into a dead, monotonous routine, do whatever it takes to get out. If you do not value your life enough, no one else will.

- Don't sulk that you have drawn a short straw: if you do your bit, the universe will do its bit. But if you don't, you should not expect the universe to stop, reverse its course and start paying attention. It has other priorities, I assure you.

- Develop and trust your intuition: in terms of evolution, your gut has been around for a lot longer than your brain. Learn to listen to your body, and do not ignore what you hear.

- Move your body, make your heart work at pumping blood, and enjoy your physiology. If you avoid mirrors and switch the light off in the bedroom before your partner has had a chance to enjoy the look of your body, you definitely need to do something about it!

MAKE SURE YOU HAVE DAILY BOWEL MOVEMENTS.....

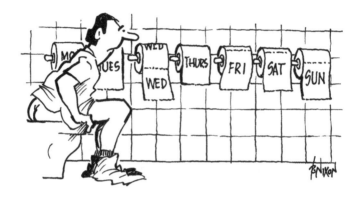

- And, of course, make sure you have daily bowel movements.

Summary: your road map to healthy living

To sum it all up, healthy living is a system that nourishes your body, your mind and your emotions and that enables you to grow. It is a foundation of a full and rewarding life.

Any system that you devise for yourself has to be sustainable in the long term, and flexible enough to reflect the changes in your life. Whatever system you select, you can't go wrong if you include the tips below:

- *Practice conscious breathing.* Use deep breathing as a

relaxation and stress management technique. Exercise your lungs daily, and make sure your skin, hair and nails also get a change to breathe every day.

• *Keep yourself hydrated.* Make sure your diet includes enough liquid, and remember that neither sweet drinks nor coffee or regular tea count towards your water intake.

As a rule of thumb, your weight in pound divided by 2 equals the number of ounces of water you need to consume in a day. So, if you weigh about 140 pounds, you need 70 ounces, and even more if you exercise, if you are ill or in hot weather.

• *Nourish your emotions.* Healthy emotions are one of the most important ingredients of healthy digestion. Life can be pretty tough, and it often is. But you *choose to* either feel like you are a victim of bad luck, or proactively change the things you can change, accepting the ones you can't.

• *Lymphasize.* Healthy lymph equals healthy immune system. Remember that, unlike blood, lymph does not have its own pressure and that it needs cellular exercise to keep moving. Rebounding, contrast showers, vibration and lymph drainage massages are some of the most common methods of lymphasizing.

• *Exercise.* Exercise works a lot better when you are positively motivated: it is much more fun to exercise to gain energy and confidence, rather than just lose weight. Use every opportunity to get your heart rate up - walk to work whenever you can, go for walks in the morning or drop in to a class on a regular basis. Find a sport that helps you grow.

• *Eat living foods.* Avoid putting into your body non-descript manufactured products. Make sure that any dietary system that you choose includes a lot of foods that have high energy and have been grown, reared and prepared with love and respect. Remember, your body will judge you by what you put into it.

• *Cleanse.* Living a clean life means living the life to the highest standard that you have set for yourself. It means that you keep growing, learning and sharing. Make sure you make conscious choices in life and that you get the most out of every day.

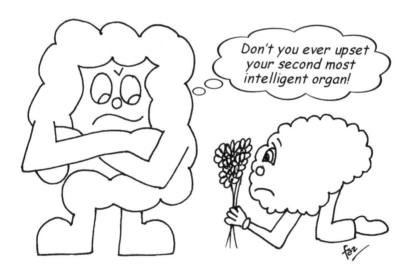

And of course, have daily bowel movements.

EPILOGUE

This journey has come to its end. Although I don't know you, I hope you have found my book useful. If you've read this far, you will probably wonder, out of natural curiosity, what my own life is like and whether I walk my talk, how I plan my own nutrition, whether I have colonics and what drives me in general.

Well... I am 46 years old. Despite having a grown-up son, I don't feel my age. I am an out-and-out townie: I live with my husband and my black cat in a town house in the town centre in Maidenhead, Berkshire, UK, within walking distance of Wellbeing Now, as well as of a park, a good book store, a great food store, an Italian deli, the railway station, the town library and a good coffee shop.

My passion

For most of my life I have been an educator: I started teaching when I was seventeen.

I strongly believe that everyone deserves a great life, and that learning and knowledge become the keys that open a lot of doors. That is why I am so passionate about sharing my knowledge with my clients and students, and helping them to grow.

I am also convinced that every few years I need to shed my skin, like a snake, and go and learn something completely new. My life gets a pretty thorough makeover about every seven years, so I don't really have the time to get bored.

Becoming an adult learner, I have found, makes me feel vulnerable and teaches humility. But it also helps me stay young, both physically and mentally.

My diet and exercise

I am a natural raw food eater, and during the warm English season, raw food probably constitutes about 80% to 85% of my diet. In winter I mostly eat soups and warm salads.

I do not eat any processed food at home, and try to avoid it whenever I travel.

I don't do any strenuous exercise, but I often walk to work, go for morning walks, and do rebounding, yoga and stretching. My mind never stops working, and I have to force myself to slow down and meditate.

My favourite dish is a salad made with rocket and beetroot leaves, home-grown sprouts, avocados, buffalo mozzarella, virgin olive oil, lemon and balsamic vinegar.

My healthy drinks of choice are freshly squeezed vegetable and fruit juices and kefir, which I make at home from goat's milk and kefir culture.

I wouldn't describe myself as a nutritional sinner. My 'pleasure islands' are a double espresso, a good glass of wine and an occasional portion of organic dark chocolate ice cream, eaten with a spoon straight out of the carton while I am watching a movie.

Bodywork and colonics

I love giving and receiving treatments. My favourite treatments are sports massage, body wraps, and, as you have probably guessed, colonics.

I have several colonics a year, but generally no more than three or four, unless I am under huge stress or need an immunity boost.

As I travel a lot, both for work and pleasure, I make sure I taste different treatments from different world cultures. I love the sensuality and energy of human touch.

Every time I get upset or angry, all I need to do is remember some of the great treatments I have had: an incredible two-hour water massage in Blue Lagoon in Reykjavik, an amazing fruit body wrap under a waterfall in Fiji, or a deep pressure massage in Seoul, after which I floated above humanity for about a week.

Generally, I am a happy person. I make sure my life has pleasure in it, and this is both my insurance policy and my energy bank. I have a great relationship with my husband, I love my family. I share my love and knowledge with people, and they share theirs with me.

At the end of the day, that's what it is all about.

The books that will take you on more journeys

THE BOOKS THAT WILL TAKE YOU ON MORE JOURNEYS.....

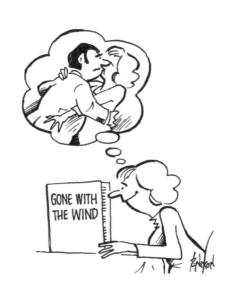

THE BOOKS THAT WILL TAKE YOU ON MORE JOURNEYS

Introduction

Books are vessels that travel the world to deliver thoughts.

No one single book can deliver everything, especially if we are dealing with such a comprehensive, all-embracing phenomenon as healthy living.

My 'vessel' has covered a very small aspect of healthy living - bowel eliminations and the connections between the eliminations and your health. It has also shown you how to use colonic irrigation as a tool to enhance your digestive health and general wellbeing.

There are many, many more books that you can read if you are interested in other aspects of your physical, emotional or mental health.

The books listed below are some of the many books that have helped me start to understand the human body, to improve my health, to teach my students, and to educate my clients and so on. I hope these books will help you continue your journey of self-discovery.

The book list

Optimal Digestion - New Strategies for Achieving Digestive Health
Edited by Trent W. Nichols, MD, and Nancy Faass, MSW, MPH
ISBN: 0-38080-498-0 (A)

The Second Brain
By Michael D. Gershon, MD
ISBN: 0-06093-072-1 (A)

The Nutritional Health Handbook for Women
By Dr Marilyn Glenville PhD
ISBN: 0 7499 2235 4 PBK

Women's Bodies, Women's Wisdom
By Dr Christiane Northrup
ISBN: 0-74991-925-6 (A)

Brain Longevity
By Dharma Singh Khalsa MD
ISBN: 0-44652-067-5 (A)

Creating Health
By Deepak Chopra
ISBN: 1-84413-565-9

Energy Secrets, the Ultimate Well-Being Plan
By Alla Svirinskaya
ISBN: 1-40190-630-3 (A)

Your Body's Many Cries for Water
By F. Batmanghelidj, MD
ISBN: 0-96299-423-5

Spiritual Nutrition
By Dr Gabriel Cousens, MD
ISBN: 1-55643-499-5 (A)

You Are What You Eat
By Dr Gillian McKeith
ISBN: 0-71814-765-0 (A)

Chi-Gung. Harnessing the Power of the Universe
By Daniel Reid
ISBN: 0-68482-125-7

Dr Bob Arnot's Revolutionary Weight Control Program
By Robert Arnot, MD
ISBN: 0-31605-167-5 (A)

Living Yoga
By Ernest Coates
ISBN: 0-95291-820-X

Smart Exercise - Burning Fat, Getting Fit
By Covert Bailey
ISBN: 0-39566-114-5 (A)

The Juice Master: Turbo-charge your life in 14 days
By Jason Vale
ISBN: 0 00 719422 6

Colonic Questionnaire
used in Wellbeing Now

Wellbeing Now
17 North Town Road Maidenhead Berks SL6 7JQ
Tel: 01628 - 670 - 970

Web: www.wellbeingnow.co.uk   Email: request@wellbeingnow.co.uk

Colonic Irrigation Questionnaire - Please fill this questionnaire and bring it with you to your treatment.

Surname:		Sex:		Have you had colonics before: Y N
Name:		Age:		What therapies do you use regularly?
Telephone No:		Weight:		
Mobile:		E-Mail:		

Reasons for the treatment (tick the ones that apply to you):

Kick-start healthy living	Irregular bowel movements	Lack of energy	Skin problems
Detox	Constipation	Food cravings	Allergies
Increase energy	IBS/Bloatedness	Mood swings	Parasites
Help with weight loss	Diarrhoea	Yeasts/Candida	Headaches/migraines

Have these conditions lasted: over 1-year   2-3 years   5 years or longer

Tick the statements that apply to your eating habits and lifestyle:

I have a balanced diet ☐	I smoke & drink ☐	I snack on sweets/chocolate ☐
I drink 8 glasses of water/day ☐	I chew thoroughly ☐	I often overeat ☐
I don't take milk		
I don't eat wheat		
I exercise enough ☐	I eat quickly ☐	I have big meals after 8 pm ☐
I eat salads/vegetables		
I do not exercise enough ☐	I eat ready meals ☐	I often eat bread, pasta etc ☐
I eat rice, barley etc		

217

Please state your occupation and describe the levels of stress, *a typical workday eating pattern*, including meals, snacks and liquid intake. If you smoke or drink alcohol *please state how much. If you take recreational drugs please mention this to the practitioner.*

Describe your typical bowel movements: frequency, amounts and appearance

Please check whether you have any of the following conditions for which this treatment is contraindicated:

☐ Severe Cardiac Disease ☐ Severe Anaemia ☐ Active fissures/fistulae ☐ Recent colorectal surgery ☐ Cirrhosis or abd. hernia
☐ Unmonitored High BP ☐ GI haemmorage/perf ☐ Pregnancy 1st trimestre ☐ Renal insufficiency ☐ Colorectal carcinoma

Please check if you have had any of the following:

☐ Cancer ☐ Diabetes ☐ High Blood Pressure ☐ Heart Disease ☐ Hepatitis
☐ Rheumatic Fever ☐ Thyroid Disease ☐ Seizures ☐ Other

Please add any information on operations/surgeries in the last 5 years (continue on the reverse if needed):

Please list any Medications and Nutritional Supplements you take on a daily basis (continue on the reverse if needed):

Please sign and date this questionnaire.
By signing this form I accept the 'Terms and Conditions of Booking' printed on the advice & reference page

Signature: Date:

USEFUL RESOURCES

The website of "Always look after Number Two":
www.colonicbook.com

Colon hydrotherapy associations:
International Association of Colon Therapists (I-ACT):
www.i-act.org

The Association of Registered Colon Hydrotherapists
(ARCH): www.colonic-association.org

Colon hydrotherapy training
(I-ACT instructors and curriculum)

The Chi Centre
17 North Town Road
Maidenhead, SL6 7JQ
United Kingdom

www.wellbeingnow.co.uk
www.detoxbreaks.co.uk
www.healingbreaks.co.uk

Shopping:
www.healthybuys.co.uk

Useful health-related websites:

Womens' Health
www.marilynglenville.com

Juicing and exercise:
www.thejuicemaster.com

Nutrition and nutritional education:
www.ion.ac.uk

MY USEFUL RESOURCES

Exercise routine for stress and tension relief, bowel support & digestive health

I am very grateful to Ernest Coates, a modern Yoga guru and past chairman of Friends of Yoga International, for allowing me the use of his text and illustrations in this exercise routine.

It is based on a more detailed description of these exercises in Ernest Coates' Living Yoga (ISBN: 0-95291-820-X).

It is recommended to perform this routine with someone more experienced or a teacher for the first couple of times, till you are confident that you are exercising in the right way.

This routine needs to be performed daily, or at least every other day, to achieve effectiveness.

Disclaimer

As with any exercise programme, if you are unsure whether this practice would be beneficial for you, please consult a fitness and health professional or your doctor.

Have a great workout!

Background notes and useful reminders

According to ancient teaching, all functions of the body are controlled by phlegm, wind and bile, known as humours.

The wind is not only gastric and intestinal gases but also the wind formed in every joint due to chemical reactions causing rheumatic pains and stiffness. The acid and bile associated with the digestive juices, as well as the uric acid, need to be eliminated from the body in order to stop excessive acidity from affecting some organs and parts of the body.

This routine is useful for everyone suffering from stress, tension and digestive discomfort, as well as for people recovering from illness, or those who have muscular problems.

These exercises are also beneficial for those experiencing muscle and joint stiffness.

The series of exercises below can be divided into two sections:

- The tension release (anti-rheumatic group), in exercises 1 to 20;

- The gas and toxic release group, in exercises 21 to 30.

Ideally, these exercises should be performed in the order given.

To help remember the routine of the tension release exercises, remember to start at the toes and work up the body exercise by exercise, to the neck.

After the exercises can be performed comfortably, attention can be given to the breath.

As a general guide, you should:

- Breathe in while lifting any part of the body or back bending backwards; and

- Breathe out lowering any part of the body or bending forwards.

Please follow more detailed breathing instructions given with specific exercises below.

It is essential to focus and be very aware of the body part being exercised. Think of toes, or feet, or ankles, etc, and do not let the mind wander. If it does, bring the mind back every time.

The positions included in this book can be performed at any time of the day and will help relieve the day's stress, release tension, massage organs and glands, relax the nerves and help to bring about a more tranquil mental state.

Adapted from Living Yoga by Ernest Coates

"Rep" stands for "repetitions"

TENSION RELEASE AND
ANTI-RHEUMATIC EXERCISES

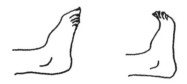

Exercise 1 - Toe Bending

(5-10 reps each foot)

Sit on the mat with your legs stretched, keeping both feet straight pointing upwards. Bend the toes backwards and forwards.

Exercise 2 - feet Bending

(5-10 reps each foot)

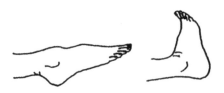

From the same position, stretch the feet forwards and down, then up and backwards as far as possible.

Exercise 3 - Ankle Rotation

(5-10 reps clockwise and anticlockwise for each ankle)

From the same position, place the right ankle on top of the left thigh and grasp the toes with the left hand, rotating the foot clockwise, then anti-clockwise. The right hand can rest and hold the right knee. Repeat the other leg.

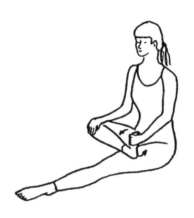

Exercise 4 - Knee Bending

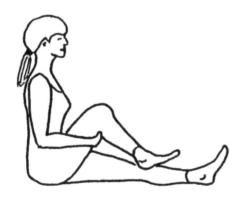

(5-10 reps each leg)

From the same position, hold under the right thigh with both hands. Bend the right leg and bring the heel close to the buttock. Now straighten the right leg without touching the floor. Repeat 5 - 10 times, then do the other leg.

Exercise 5 - Half-Butterfly

(10-20 reps each leg)

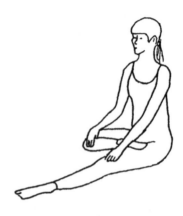

Staying in the same position, bend the right leg and place the foot on the left thigh. Place the right hand on top of the right knee and gently push the leg down trying to touch the floor with the right knee. Keep the leg straight with the left hand on top or holding the right foot.

Exercise 6 - Butterfly

(10-20 reps)

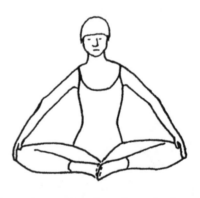

Bend both legs, place the soles of the feet together. Interlace the fingers under the feet or over the toes and pull the heels as close to the body as possible. Now gently push the knees to the floor. The elbows can be used to push the knees down or the hands can be placed on the knees to push them down, allowing the knees to return upwards each time. A more difficult stage is to bend forward trying to lower the head to the floor while pushing the knees down.

Exercise 7 - Crow Walking

(30 secs - 2 min)

Squat with the palms on the knees and walk in this position, either on feet or toes. A more difficult variation is to touch the floor with the knee each time a step is taken. This is a very good leg exercise that also improves circulation in the legs and remedies constipation.

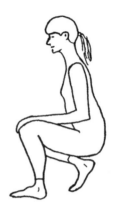

Exercise 8 - Lower Spine Stretch

(5-10 reps)

From the seated position, raise both arms to the horizontal straight in front with

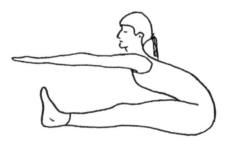

the hands pointing to the feet. Keep the head back, stretch forward, focusing on the lower back.

Exercise 9 - *Spinal Stretch*

(5-10 reps)

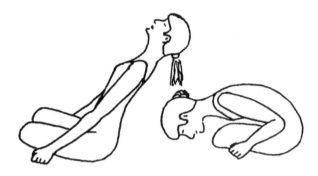

Sit cross legged with the hands holding the feet, arch the back, then bend forward to bring the head to the floor in front of the crossed legs.

Exercise 10 - *Spinal Twist*

(5-10 rounds)

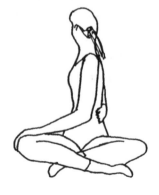

Sit cross-legged, place the left hand on the right knee, turn the head and trunk to the right looking behind as far as possible, and at the same time, bend the right arm behind the back and place the right palm against the left waist. Twist the spine as far as possible then repeat in the opposite direction to complete one round.

Exercise 11 - Hand Clenching

(5-10 reps)

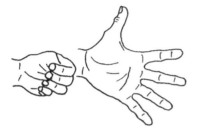

Sitting on the mat with the arms straight out in front, stretch and tense the fingers or both hands then make fists with both hands. Repeat 5 - 10 times.

Exercise 12 - Wrist Bending

(10-20 reps)

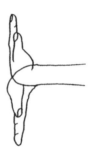

From the above position, bend the hands at the wrist, pointing the fingers upwards then downwards. Repeat 5 -10 times.

Exercise 13 - Wrist Rotation

(5-10 reps clockwise and anticlockwise for each wrist)

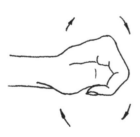

In the same position by with only the right arm extended in front, make a fist and rotate it clockwise then anti-clockwise. Repeat with the other hand.

Exercise 14 - Elbow Bending

(10-20 reps)

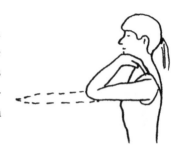

From the same position with the arms in front and the hands facing up, bend both arms and wrists and touch the shoulders with the fingers, then straighten the arms.

Exercise 15 - Shoulder Rotation

(5-10 reps clockwise and anticlockwise for each shoulder)

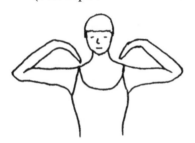

In the same position, with the arms and wrists bent and the fingers touching the shoulders, rotate the arms from the shoulders, making a circular movement with each elbow as large as possible. The elbows should contact each other in front of the chest and the fingers should keep in contact with the shoulders.

Exercise 16 - Shoulder Shrug

(5-10 reps forward and backward for each shoulder)

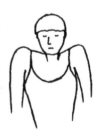

From the same position, shrug the shoulders up and forwards and then up and backwards.

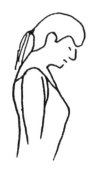

Exercise 17 - Neck, Forward and Back

(3-6 reps)

In a seated position, slowly lower the head, chin to chest, then raise the head and stretch the throat.

Exercise 18 - Neck, Side Stretch

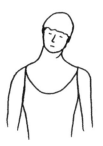

(3-6 rounds)

Slowly lower the head to the left (left ear to left shoulder) looking ahead, then straighten the head and lower the right side.

Exercise 19 - Neck Turning

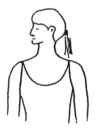

(3-6 rounds)

Slowly turn the head to the left, then to the right.

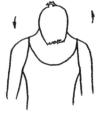

Exercise 20 - Head Rotation

(3-6 rounds)

Slowly rotate the head, making as large a circle as possible.

GAS AND TOXIC RELEASE EXERCISES

These exercises remove wind and gas from the stomach and intestines. They help alleviate indigestion and constipation and are useful in overcoming neuromuscular problems.

Exercise 21 - Leg Rotation

(5-10 reps - clockwise and anticlockwise for each leg)

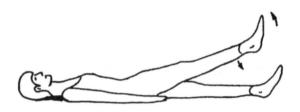

Lie on the back with the arms close to the body, palms pressed down to the floor. Raise the right leg off the floor and rotate in a clockwise direction , then in an anti-clockwise direction. Repeat with the left leg, and then relax. The exercise can be repeated with both legs together.

Exercise 22 - Cycling, One Leg

5-10 reps clockwise and anticlockwise for each leg)

From the same position, raise the right leg to the vertical, cycle forwards, and then reverse cycle movements. Repeat with the other leg.

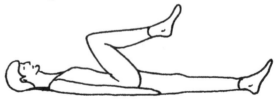

Exercise 23 - Cycling, Alternate Legs

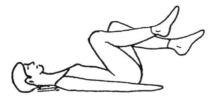

(5-10 rounds clockwise and anticlockwise)

From the same position perform alternative leg forward cycling movements, then in reverse. Make sure your lower back is pressing down into the mat.

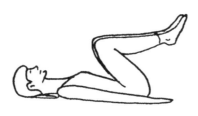

Exercise 24 - Cycling, Both Legs

(5-10 rounds clockwise and anticlockwise)

Keeping both legs together, cycle forward, and then back. Make sure your lower back is pressing down into the mat.

Exercise 25 - Head to Each Knee

(5 reps each leg)

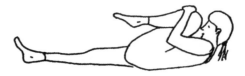

Lie on the back and bend the right leg to the chest. Breathing in, interlace the fingers over the knee and breathe out, now raise the head and upper part of the body to touch the knee with the chin or nose. Breathe in and return to lying on the back.

Exercise 26 - Head to Knees

(5-10 reps)

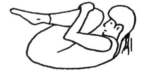

Bend both legs to the chest and wrap both arms around the knees, breathing in. Raise the head to the knees breathing out.

Exercise 27 - Rolling

(5-10 rounds)

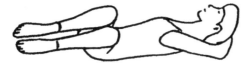

From the above position, roll the body sideways from one side to the other 5 - 10 times.

Alternatively the fingers can be interlaced behind the head with the knees bent to the chest and the rolling motion done keeping the elbows to the floor.

Exercise 28 - Rocking

(5-10 rounds)

From the position with the knees bent and the arms around the knees, rock the body backwards and forwards so as to massage the back. Try to reach a squatting position on the forward movement and take care when rocking back to avoid the head hitting the ground hard.

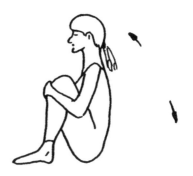

Exercise 29 - Sit-ups

(5 reps)

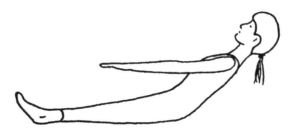

Lie on the back with the arms above the head. Breathe in and raise the trunk to about 30 degrees off the floor, bring the arms up and over to point the hands to the feet. Breathe out and lower back to the floor.

Exercise 30 - Boat

(5 reps)

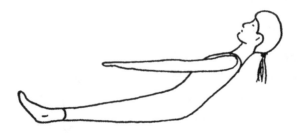

Lie on the back with the arms close to the body, palms down. Breathe in and raise the legs, arms, trunk and head off the floor, the arms to be parallel to the floor, breathe out and lower to the floor. During the last round hold the breath in the raised position, tensing the body. Breathe out and lower to the floor and relax.

To finish off the exercises, lie down on the mat and stretch with your arms fully extended behind your back and the eyes closed, restoring your breathing.

While you are resting, keep your mind focused on the positive feelings that your body is experiencing: relaxation, balance and peace.

If your mind starts wandering, catch it and bring it back into the body.

Scan your body, from the feet up. Thank it silently for coping with all the stresses that you go through and for being there for you every single minute.

Remember, your body is the home where all your thoughts, feelings and emotions come to stay. Look after your home, because you won't get another one!

My personal wellbeing plan

My personal wellbeing plan

My personal wellbeing plan

My personal wellbeing plan

Always Look After Number Two!

Order Form

Email: request@colonicbook.com

Postal Order: Please fill in the form below and return to
                Fotherby Press
                c/o Wellbeing Now, 17 North Town Road,
                Maidenhead, Berks SL6 7JQ, UK

Please send me more free information on:

☐ Speaking/Seminars ☐ Training ☐ Consulting ☐ Trade orders

Please note that UK orders can only be delivered to the cardholder's address. If you require delivery to a different address please pay by cheque or on line at www.colonicbook.com

Name: _____

Address: _____

City: _____ County: _____

Post/Zip Code: _____ Country: _____

Contact Number: (inc. area code) _____

Email Address: _____

Always Look After Number Two! Price per copy: £9.99	Qty	Total Price
Total for books		£
Postage & Packing (UK)		£
Postage & Packing (Int)		£
Total Amount Enclosed		£

Payment Type: ☐ Cheque (payable to Fotherby Press- UK £'s only)

☐ Credit Card   ☐ Debit Card   ☐ Mastercard   ☐ Visa

Card No: _____

Valid from: _____ Valid to: _____ Issue No: _____

Signature: _____

Please note: photocopied signatures cannot be accepted

Postage, Packing & Handling Charges:

Delivery UK & Europe

1-4 books - £1.85 per book, 5 and more - £0.75 per book

Rest of the world:

1-4 books - £3.50 per book, 5 and more - £2.50 per book